THE ANTI-INFLAMMATORY LIFESTYLE DIET COOKBOOK

Nourishing Recipes and Meal Plans to Reduce Inflammation, Promote Healing, and Optimize Wellness

Grace Mitchell

Table of Content

INTRODUCTION 10

    Understanding Inflammation and Its Impact on Health 10

    Benefits of an Anti-Inflammatory Diet 11

FOUNDATIONS OF AN ANTI-INFLAMMATORY DIET 13

    Key Principles and Guidelines 13

    Foods to Include and Avoid 16

ESSENTIAL KITCHEN TOOLS AND INGREDIENTS 20

    Essential Kitchen Tools: 20

    Essential Ingredients: 22

MEAL PLANNING AND PREP TIPS 26

    Batch Cooking and Freezing Techniques 26

    Creating Balanced Meals 28

    Tips for Grocery Shopping 30

BREAKFAST IDEAS 36

    Berry Spinach Smoothie Bowl 36

    Overnight Oats with Blueberries and Chia Seeds 38

    Turmeric and Ginger Smoothie 40

    Quinoa Breakfast Porridge 42

    Chia Pudding with Mango and Coconut 44

    Green Detox Smoothie 46

Oatmeal with Flaxseeds and Berries 48

Avocado Toast with Cherry Tomatoes and Basil 50

Sweet Potato Hash with Spinach and Eggs 52

Spinach and Mushroom Egg Muffins..54

Banana Almond Butter Toast..56

Pumpkin Spice Smoothie 57

Coconut Almond Granola..59

LUNCH AND DINNER RECIPES 61

Grilled Salmon with Quinoa and Asparagus 61

Lentil and Vegetable Stew 63

Turmeric Roasted Cauliflower and Chickpeas 65

Roasted Butternut Squash and Kale Salad..67

Zucchini Noodles with Pesto and Cherry Tomatoes 69

Spinach and Mushroom Quinoa 71

Thai Chicken Lettuce Wraps 73

Garlic Lemon Shrimp with Zoodles 75

Stuffed Portobello Mushrooms 77

Chicken and Vegetable Stir-Fry...79

Baked Cod with Sweet Potato and Brussels Sprouts 81

Mediterranean Chickpea Salad 83

Quinoa and Black Bean Tacos 85

SNACKS AND APPETIZERS 87

Guacamole with Veggie Sticks 87

Roasted Chickpeas 88

Hummus with Cucumber Slices 90

Baked Sweet Potato Fries 91

Trail Mix with Nuts and Dried Fruit 93

Edamame with Sea Salt 94

Apple Slices with Almond Butter 95

Greek Yogurt with Berries and Honey 96

Carrot and Celery Sticks with Tahini Dip..97

Stuffed Dates with Almonds...99

Kale Chips...100

Berry and Nut Energy Balls 101

Avocado Deviled Eggs 102

Quinoa and Veggie Bites 104

SAUCES, DRESSINGS, AND DIPS 106

Classic Hummus...106

Avocado Cilantro Dressing..107

Turmeric Tahini Sauce 109

Lemon Vinaigrette... 110

Pesto Sauce...112

Cucumber Dill Dip...113

Spicy Peanut Sauce..115

Mango Salsa 116

Garlic Herb Aioli 118

Cashew Cream 119

Chimichurri Sauce...120

Honey Mustard Dressing 122

Ginger Miso Dressing 123

Coconut Curry Sauce 124

DESSERTS AND SWEET TREATS...................................... 126

Dark Chocolate Avocado Mousse 126

Coconut Macaroons...127

Banana Ice Cream 129

Almond Flour Brownies 130

Berry Crumble 132

Pumpkin Pie Energy Balls 134

Baked Apples with Cinnamon 136

Matcha Green Tea Energy Bites 138

Peanut Butter and Dark Chocolate Bark 140

Lemon Coconut Bliss Balls 142

Raspberry Chia Jam Bars 144

Mango Sorbet 146

Coconut Yogurt with Fresh Fruit....................................148

Blueberry Oat Muffins...149

BEVERAGES AND SMOOTHIES 151

Green Detox Smoothie 151

Turmeric Golden Milk 152

Berry Banana Smoothie 154

Coconut Water with Lime and Mint 155

Matcha Latte...156

Ginger Lemon Tea 158

Pumpkin Spice Smoothie 159

Mango Pineapple Smoothie 160

Avocado Spinach Smoothie 162

Chia Seed Lemonade 163

Apple Cinnamon Smoothie 164

Beetroot and Berry Smoothie 166

Cucumber Mint Cooler 167

Papaya Ginger Smoothie 168

Watermelon Basil Cooler 170

GLUTEN-FREE OPTIONS 172

Quinoa and Black Bean Salad 172

Cauliflower Rice Stir-Fry 174

Stuffed Bell Peppers 176

Baked Salmon with Asparagus 178

Lentil and Vegetable Soup 180

Grilled Chicken with Quinoa and Veggies 182

Spinach and Mushroom Frittata 184

Shrimp and Zoodle Stir-Fry 186

Roasted Butternut Squash Salad 188

Chicken Lettuce Wraps 190

Coconut Curry Chicken 192

Mediterranean Chickpea Salad 194

VEGAN AND VEGETARIAN VARIATIONS 196

Chickpea and Avocado Salad 196

Quinoa Stuffed Bell Peppers 197

Lentil and Spinach Stew 200

Vegan Mushroom Stroganoff 202

Zucchini Noodles with Marinara Sauce 204

Tofu and Vegetable Stir-Fry 206

Baked Falafel with Tahini Sauce 208

Vegan Buddha Bowl 210

Cauliflower Tacos 213

Vegan Lentil Loaf 216

Roasted Veggie Power Bowl 218

Vegan Pumpkin Curry 221

Vegan Black Bean Burgers 223

LIFESTYLE TIPS 226

Incorporating Exercise 226

Stress Management 228

Ensuring Quality Sleep 229

TIPS FOR DINING OUT AND SOCIAL EVENTS...................................232

Tips for Dining Out 232

Tips for Social Events 234

Strategies for Travel and Holidays 236

Building Resilience and Flexibility...237

INCORPORATING MINDFUL EATING PRACTICES 239

Principles of Mindful Eating 239

Tips for Incorporating Mindful Eating Practices 240

Benefits of Mindful Eating 243

CONCLUSION 245

30-Days Anti-Inflammatory Meal Plan 247

INTRODUCTION

Welcome to "The Anti-Inflammatory Lifestyle Diet Cookbook: Nourishing Recipes and Meal Plans to Reduce Inflammation, Promote Healing, and Optimize Wellness." Whether you're dealing with chronic inflammation or simply seeking a healthier lifestyle, this book is your companion on a journey to better health. Here, you'll find delicious recipes, practical meal plans, and the knowledge you need to make informed dietary choices that can transform your life.

Anti-inflammatory eating isn't just a diet—it's a lifestyle. It's about embracing foods that support your body's natural defenses and reducing those that can trigger inflammation. This book aims to make this transition easy and enjoyable, with recipes that are as tasty as they are nourishing. As you turn these pages, you'll discover that eating to reduce inflammation doesn't mean sacrificing flavor or joy in your meals. Instead, you'll find a vibrant way to eat that nourishes your body and soul.

Understanding Inflammation and Its Impact on Health

Inflammation is your body's natural response to injury or infection. It's like an internal alarm system, signaling your immune system to spring into action. In small doses, inflammation is a healing force. But when it becomes chronic, it can turn against you, leading to a host of health problems.

Imagine a fire that never fully extinguishes. It smolders and spreads, affecting different parts of your body. This chronic inflammation is linked to various diseases, including heart disease, diabetes, arthritis, and even depression. It can leave you feeling constantly fatigued, in pain, and out of balance.

Understanding inflammation means recognizing the signs your body is sending you. It's about listening to your aches and pains, acknowledging persistent fatigue, and noticing the subtle shifts in your overall health. By doing so, you can take proactive steps to cool the flames and restore your well-being.

Benefits of an Anti-Inflammatory Diet

Switching to an anti-inflammatory diet offers a multitude of benefits, extending far beyond the relief of physical symptoms. Imagine waking up feeling energized, your mind clear, and your body free from pain. This diet can help make that a reality.

Firstly, you'll experience a significant reduction in chronic pain and discomfort. Foods rich in antioxidants and omega-3 fatty acids, like berries and fatty fish, work to soothe inflammation at the cellular level. You'll find that common issues like joint pain, headaches, and muscle soreness diminish.

Secondly, your energy levels will soar. Chronic inflammation often leads to chronic fatigue, but an anti-inflammatory diet fuels your body with essential nutrients, leading to sustained energy throughout the day. Whole grains, leafy greens, and nuts provide the steady energy your body needs.

Moreover, an anti-inflammatory diet supports better mental health. There's a strong connection between gut health and brain health, often referred to as the gut-brain axis. By nourishing your gut with probiotics and fiber-rich foods, you promote a healthier brain, reducing symptoms of anxiety and depression.

Additionally, this diet is a powerful ally in preventing and managing chronic diseases. By reducing inflammation, you lower your risk of heart disease, diabetes, and even certain cancers. It's a proactive approach to long-term health and longevity.

Finally, the anti-inflammatory diet is not about restriction but about abundance. You'll explore a diverse array of foods that are both nutritious and delicious. From colorful vegetables to exotic spices, every meal becomes an adventure in taste and health.

As you embark on this journey, remember that change doesn't happen overnight. Be patient with yourself, celebrate small victories, and enjoy the process of discovering a healthier, happier you. This book is here to guide you every step of the way, offering practical advice, inspiring recipes, and the encouragement you need to succeed.

Welcome to a life of vibrant health and wellness. Welcome to the anti-inflammatory way of living.

FOUNDATIONS OF AN ANTI-INFLAMMATORY DIET

Changing your connection with food is as important as altering your diet when starting an anti-inflammatory diet. You will learn the fundamental ideas and rules in this chapter, which will help you make this transition seamless and long-lasting.

Key Principles and Guidelines

1. Embrace Whole, Unprocessed Foods

The cornerstone of an anti-inflammatory diet is whole, unprocessed foods. These foods are as close to their natural state as possible, free from additives, preservatives, and artificial ingredients. Whole foods include fruits, vegetables, whole grains, nuts, seeds, and lean proteins. They are nutrient-dense, providing your body with essential vitamins, minerals, and antioxidants that fight inflammation.

2. Prioritize Plant-Based Eating

While an anti-inflammatory diet doesn't require you to be vegetarian or vegan, it emphasizes plant-based eating. Plants are rich in phytonutrients—natural compounds with anti-inflammatory properties. Aim to fill at least half of your plate with fruits and vegetables at each meal. Leafy greens, berries, tomatoes, and cruciferous vegetables like broccoli and cauliflower are particularly potent in reducing inflammation.

3. Choose Healthy Fats

Not all fats are created equal. Healthy fats, such as those found in olive oil, avocados, nuts, and fatty fish, can help reduce inflammation. These fats are rich in omega-3 fatty acids, which are known for their anti-inflammatory benefits. On the other hand, trans fats and saturated fats, often found in processed and fried foods, can exacerbate inflammation and should be limited.

4. Opt for Lean Proteins

Protein is essential for repairing tissues and maintaining muscle mass, but the type of protein you choose matters. Lean proteins such as chicken, turkey, fish, beans, and legumes are excellent choices. Fatty fishes like salmon, mackerel, and sardines are especially beneficial due to their high omega-3 content. Reducing red meat and processed meats, which can increase inflammation, is also advisable.

5. Reduce Sugar and Refined Carbohydrates

Excessive sugar and refined carbohydrates, found in sugary drinks, pastries, white bread, and many packaged snacks, can trigger inflammation. These foods cause spikes in blood sugar levels, leading to an inflammatory response. Instead, opt for complex carbohydrates such as whole grains, brown rice, quinoa, and sweet potatoes, which provide sustained energy and have a lower impact on blood sugar.

6. Stay Hydrated

Hydration plays a crucial role in maintaining your body's functions and reducing inflammation. Water helps to flush out toxins and supports overall cellular health. Aim to drink at least eight 8-ounce glasses of water a day, and consider incorporating herbal teas and water-rich fruits and vegetables like cucumbers and watermelon.

7. Spice It Up

Herbs and spices are not only flavorful additions to your meals but also powerful anti-inflammatory agents. Turmeric, ginger, garlic, cinnamon, and cayenne pepper have been shown to reduce inflammation and provide numerous health benefits. Incorporate these spices into your cooking to enhance both the taste and the health benefits of your meals.

8. Practice Mindful Eating

Mindful eating involves paying attention to what and how you eat. Slow down, savor each bite, and listen to your body's hunger and fullness cues. This practice can help you make more conscious food choices and improve your digestion and overall relationship with food.

Foods to Include and Avoid

Understanding which foods to include and avoid is crucial for following an anti-inflammatory diet effectively. Here's a detailed guide to help you make informed choices:

Foods to Include

1. **Fruits and Vegetables**:
   - **Berries** (blueberries, strawberries, raspberries): Rich in antioxidants.
   - **Leafy Greens** (spinach, kale, Swiss chard): High in vitamins and minerals.
   - **Cruciferous Vegetables** (broccoli, Brussels sprouts, cauliflower): Contain anti-inflammatory compounds.
   - **Tomatoes**: Packed with lycopene, which has anti-inflammatory properties.

2. **Whole Grains**:
   - **Quinoa**: A complete protein with anti-inflammatory benefits.
   - **Brown Rice**: A fiber-rich alternative to white rice.
   - **Oats**: Contain beta-glucan, which reduces inflammation.

3. **Healthy Fats**:
   - **Olive Oil**: Rich in monounsaturated fats and antioxidants.
   - **Avocados**: High in healthy fats and fiber.
   - **Nuts and Seeds** (almonds, chia seeds, flaxseeds): Provide omega-3 fatty acids and other nutrients.

4. **Lean Proteins**:
   - **Fatty Fish** (salmon, mackerel, sardines): Excellent sources of omega-3 fatty acids.
   - **Poultry** (chicken, turkey): Lean sources of protein.
   - **Legumes** (beans, lentils): High in fiber and protein.

5. **Herbs and Spices**:
   - **Turmeric**: Contains curcumin, a potent anti-inflammatory compound.
   - **Ginger**: Known for its anti-inflammatory and digestive benefits.
   - **Garlic**: Contains sulfur compounds that have anti-inflammatory effects.

6. **Beverages**:
   - **Green Tea**: High in antioxidants, particularly epigallocatechin gallate (EGCG).
   - **Herbal Teas** (ginger tea, turmeric tea): Anti-inflammatory and soothing.

Foods to Avoid

1. **Sugary Foods and Beverages**:
   - **Soda**: High in sugar and artificial ingredients.
   - **Candy and Pastries**: Loaded with refined sugars and unhealthy fats.
   - **Sugary Cereals**: Often contain high levels of sugar and low nutritional value.

2. **Refined Carbohydrates**:
   - **White Bread**: Lacks fiber and nutrients.
   - **White Rice**: Less nutritious compared to brown rice and other whole grains.
   - **Pasta** (made from refined flour): Opt for whole-grain versions instead.

3. **Processed and Red Meats**:
   - **Bacon**: High in saturated fats and additives.
   - **Sausages**: Often contain preservatives and unhealthy fats.
   - **Hot Dogs**: Processed meats with added chemicals.

4. **Trans Fats and Unhealthy Oils**:
   - **Fried Foods**: Typically fried in oils high in trans fats.
   - **Margarine**: Contains trans fats that can trigger inflammation.
   - **Vegetable Oils** (corn oil, soybean oil): High in omega-6 fatty acids, which can be inflammatory in excess.

5. **Dairy Products**:
   - **Whole Milk**: High in saturated fats.
   - **Cheese**: Can be high in saturated fats and sodium.
   - **Ice Cream**: Contains sugar and unhealthy fats.

6. **Excessive Alcohol**:
   - **Beer, Wine, and Spirits**: Can cause inflammation when consumed in excess. Moderate consumption may have some benefits, but overindulgence is harmful.

By incorporating these principles and guidelines into your daily life, you can start to reduce inflammation, improve your overall health, and enjoy a more vibrant and energetic lifestyle. The journey towards an anti-inflammatory way of eating is a rewarding one, filled with delicious foods and profound health benefits. Welcome to the foundation of your new, healthier life.

ESSENTIAL KITCHEN TOOLS AND INGREDIENTS

Cooking delicious and healthful anti-inflammatory meals doesn't require a professional kitchen setup. However, having the right tools and ingredients on hand can make the process smoother, more enjoyable, and effective. This chapter will guide you through the essential kitchen tools and ingredients needed to start your anti-inflammatory cooking journey.

Essential Kitchen Tools:

1. **Quality Knives**
   - **Chef's Knife**: A versatile knife for chopping, slicing, and dicing.
   - **Paring Knife**: Ideal for peeling and intricate tasks.
   - **Serrated Knife**: Perfect for cutting bread and tomatoes.

2. **Cutting Boards**
   - **Wooden Cutting Board**: Gentle on knives and ideal for vegetables and herbs.
   - **Plastic Cutting Board**: Suitable for raw meat and fish to avoid cross-contamination.

3. **Measuring Cups and Spoons**
   - **Dry Measuring Cups**: For measuring flour, grains, and other dry ingredients.
   - **Liquid Measuring Cups**: For measuring liquids accurately.
   - **Measuring Spoons**: Essential for spices, baking powder, and other small quantities.

4. **Mixing Bowls**
   - **Stainless Steel Bowls**: Durable and versatile for mixing and tossing salads.
   - **Glass Bowls**: Great for microwaving and serving.

5. **Cookware**
   - **Non-Stick Skillet**: Ideal for cooking with minimal oil.
   - **Cast Iron Skillet**: Excellent for even heating and high-heat cooking.
   - **Saucepan**: For making sauces, boiling grains, and simmering soups.
   - **Stockpot**: Essential for large batches of soups and stews.

6. **Baking Sheets and Pans**
   - **Baking Sheets**: For roasting vegetables and baking.
   - **Loaf Pan**: Perfect for homemade bread and meatloaf.
   - **Muffin Tin**: For portion-controlled snacks and breakfast items.

7. **Blender and Food Processor**
   - **Blender**: Essential for smoothies, soups, and sauces.
   - **Food Processor**: Great for chopping vegetables, making dough, and blending ingredients.

8. **Spatulas and Spoons**
   - **Silicone Spatula**: Heat-resistant and perfect for stirring and scraping bowls.
   - **Wooden Spoon**: Ideal for stirring soups, sauces, and stews.
   - **Slotted Spoon**: For draining and serving.

9. **Colander and Strainer**
   - **Colander**: For rinsing grains, vegetables, and draining pasta.
   - **Fine-Mesh Strainer**: Useful for straining sauces, soups, and rinsing quinoa.

10. **Storage Containers**
    - **Glass Containers**: For storing leftovers and meal prepping.
    - **Mason Jars**: Ideal for salads, dressings, and overnight oats.

11. **Zester and Grater**
    - **Microplane Zester**: Perfect for zesting citrus and grating ginger and garlic.
    - **Box Grater**: Versatile for grating cheese, vegetables, and zesting.

12. **Kitchen Scale**
    - **Digital Kitchen Scale**: For accurate measurement of ingredients, especially useful in baking and portion control.

Essential Ingredients:

1. **Fruits and Vegetables**
   - **Berries** (blueberries, strawberries, raspberries): High in antioxidants.
   - **Leafy Greens** (spinach, kale, Swiss chard): Nutrient-dense and versatile.
   - **Cruciferous Vegetables** (broccoli, Brussels sprouts, cauliflower): Rich in vitamins and anti-inflammatory compounds.

- **Root Vegetables** (sweet potatoes, carrots, beets): Great sources of fiber and vitamins.
- **Citrus Fruits** (lemons, oranges, grapefruits): Packed with vitamin C and antioxidants.

2. **Whole Grains**

- **Quinoa**: A complete protein and rich in fiber.
- **Brown Rice**: A healthy alternative to white rice.
- **Oats**: Excellent for breakfast and baking.
- **Farro and Barley**: Nutty and chewy grains great for salads and soups.

3. **Healthy Fats**

- **Olive Oil**: Rich in monounsaturated fats and antioxidants.
- **Avocado Oil**: Ideal for cooking at high temperatures.
- **Nuts and Seeds** (almonds, chia seeds, flaxseeds): Packed with omega-3 fatty acids and fiber.
- **Nut Butters** (almond butter, peanut butter): Great for snacks and smoothies.

4. **Lean Proteins**

- **Fatty Fish** (salmon, mackerel, sardines): High in omega-3 fatty acids.
- **Poultry** (chicken, turkey): Lean sources of protein.
- **Legumes** (beans, lentils, chickpeas): High in fiber and protein.
- **Tofu and Tempeh**: Plant-based protein options.

5. **Herbs and Spices**

- **Turmeric**: Contains curcumin, a powerful anti-inflammatory compound.
- **Ginger**: Known for its digestive and anti-inflammatory benefits.
- **Garlic**: Contains sulfur compounds that reduce inflammation.
- **Cinnamon**: Anti-inflammatory and adds natural sweetness.
- **Basil, Parsley, Cilantro**: Fresh herbs that enhance flavor and provide health benefits.

6. **Beverages**

- **Green Tea**: Rich in antioxidants, particularly EGCG.
- **Herbal Teas** (chamomile, ginger, turmeric): Soothing and anti-inflammatory.
- **Filtered Water**: Essential for hydration and detoxification.

7. **Pantry Staples**

- **Apple Cider Vinegar**: Known for its detoxifying properties.
- **Honey and Maple Syrup**: Natural sweeteners in moderation.
- **Tamari or Coconut Aminos**: Gluten-free alternatives to soy sauce.
- **Broth and Stock** (vegetable, chicken, beef): Base for soups and stews.
- **Canned Tomatoes**: For sauces and soups.
- **Coconut Milk**: Adds creaminess to dishes without dairy.

8. **Fermented Foods**
   - **Kimchi and Sauerkraut**: Rich in probiotics for gut health.
   - **Yogurt** (preferably non-dairy): Provides probiotics, essential for digestion.
   - **Kefir**: A fermented drink packed with probiotics.

By equipping your kitchen with these essential tools and ingredients, you'll be well-prepared to create nutritious, anti-inflammatory meals that support your health and well-being. The right tools make cooking more efficient and enjoyable, while a well-stocked pantry ensures you always have the ingredients you need to whip up a delicious and healing meal. Let's dive into the next chapters where you'll learn how to use these tools and ingredients to create mouthwatering, anti-inflammatory dishes.

MEAL PLANNING AND PREP TIPS

Effective meal planning and preparation are the backbones of a successful anti-inflammatory diet. They ensure you have nutritious meals ready to go, making it easier to stick to your healthy eating goals. This chapter will cover batch cooking and freezing techniques and guide you on how to create balanced meals that support your anti-inflammatory lifestyle.

Batch Cooking and Freezing Techniques

Batch cooking and freezing meals can save you time, reduce stress, and ensure you always have healthy options on hand. Here are some tips to help you master these techniques:

1. Plan Your Menu

- **Weekly Planning**: Dedicate time each week to plan your meals. Choose recipes that use similar ingredients to minimize waste and simplify preparation.

- **Create a Shopping List**: Write a detailed list of ingredients needed for the week. This helps you stay organized and avoid impulse buys.

2. Choose the Right Recipes

- **Freezer-Friendly Dishes**: Select recipes that freeze well, such as soups, stews, casseroles, and cooked grains.

- **Portion Control**: Opt for recipes that can be easily portioned into single servings for convenience.

3. Invest in Quality Containers

- **Glass Containers**: Use glass containers for storing cooked meals. They are durable, microwave-safe, and better for the environment.

- **Freezer Bags**: These are great for storing soups, stews, and sauces. Lay them flat in the freezer to save space.

- **Mason Jars**: Perfect for storing individual servings of salads, smoothies, and overnight oats.

4. Cooking and Cooling

- **Cook in Batches**: Prepare large quantities of food at once. For example, cook a big pot of quinoa, roast a tray of vegetables, and prepare a batch of chicken breasts.

- **Cool Properly**: Allow cooked food to cool completely before freezing. This prevents ice crystals from forming and preserves the texture and flavor of your meals.

5. Label and Date

- **Labeling**: Clearly label each container with the contents and the date it was prepared. This helps you keep track of what needs to be eaten first.

- **Rotation**: Use the oldest meals first to minimize waste and ensure freshness.

6. Freezing Techniques

- **Flash Freezing**: For individual items like berries, place them on a baking sheet and freeze until solid before transferring to a container. This prevents them from sticking together.

- **Layering**: When freezing soups or stews, leave space at the top of the container for expansion.

- **Reheating**: Thaw meals in the refrigerator overnight or use the defrost setting on your microwave. Reheat thoroughly before eating.

Creating Balanced Meals

Creating balanced meals is crucial for maintaining an anti-inflammatory diet. Balanced meals provide the right proportions of macronutrients and micronutrients, ensuring you receive comprehensive nutritional benefits.

1. Balance Your Macronutrients

- **Proteins**: Include lean proteins such as chicken, turkey, fish, legumes, tofu, and tempeh. These support muscle repair and immune function.

- **Healthy Fats**: Incorporate healthy fats from sources like olive oil, avocados, nuts, seeds, and fatty fish. These helps reduce inflammation and provide sustained energy.

- **Complex Carbohydrates**: Choose whole grains, starchy vegetables, and legumes for your carbohydrate needs. These provide fiber and steady energy.

2. Color Your Plate

- **Variety of Vegetables**: Aim for a rainbow of colors on your plate. Different colored vegetables contain various antioxidants and phytonutrients that combat inflammation.

  - **Red**: Tomatoes, bell peppers, radishes

  - **Green**: Spinach, kale, broccoli

  - **Yellow/Orange**: Carrots, sweet potatoes, squash

  - **Purple/Blue**: Eggplant, blueberries, purple cabbage

  - **White**: Cauliflower, onions, garlic

3. Portion Control

- **Vegetables**: Fill half of your plate with non-starchy vegetables. These are low in calories but high in nutrients and fiber.

- **Proteins**: Allocate a quarter of your plate to lean proteins. This helps keep you full and supports muscle health.

- **Carbohydrates**: The remaining quarter should be whole grains or starchy vegetables. These provide the necessary energy for daily activities.

4. Mindful Eating

- **Eat Slowly**: Take your time to chew and savor each bite. This aids digestion and allows your body to recognize when it's full.

- **Listen to Your Body**: Pay attention to hunger and fullness cues. Eat when you're hungry and stop when you're satisfied, not stuffed.

- **Minimize Distractions**: Focus on your meal without the distraction of screens or multitasking. This helps you enjoy your food and recognize

Tips for Grocery Shopping

Grocery shopping is a critical component of maintaining an anti-inflammatory diet. With the right strategies, you can make your shopping trips efficient, cost-effective, and focused on purchasing healthy ingredients. Here are some valuable tips to help you navigate the grocery store and make the best choices for your anti-inflammatory lifestyle:

1. Plan Ahead

Make a Shopping List

- **Organize by Sections**: Group items by categories (produce, dairy, grains) to streamline your trip.

- **Stick to Your List**: Avoid impulse buys by adhering to your planned list, ensuring you purchase only what you need.

Meal Planning

- **Weekly Menu**: Plan your meals for the week to ensure you buy all necessary ingredients.

- **Recipe Ingredients**: Check recipes for specific ingredients to avoid multiple trips to the store.

2. Shop the Perimeter

Fresh Produce

- **Fruits and Vegetables**: Load up on a variety of fresh, colorful fruits and vegetables. They are rich in antioxidants, vitamins, and minerals.

- **Leafy Greens**: Spinach, kale, and Swiss chard are excellent for salads and smoothies.

Proteins

- **Lean Meats and Fish**: Choose high-quality, lean meats like chicken, turkey, and fatty fish such as salmon.

- **Eggs and Dairy**: Opt for organic eggs and low-fat or non-dairy milk alternatives like almond or oat milk.

Healthy Fats

- **Nuts and Seeds**: Almonds, walnuts, chia seeds, and flaxseeds are great for snacking and cooking.

- **Healthy Oils**: Extra virgin olive oil and avocado oil are excellent for cooking and dressings.

3. Read Labels

Ingredients List

- **Minimal Ingredients**: Look for products with few, recognizable ingredients. Avoid items with long lists of additives and preservatives.

- **Avoid Added Sugars**: Check for hidden sugars in sauces, dressings, and snacks. Look for terms like high-fructose corn syrup, sucrose, and glucose.

Nutritional Information

- **Healthy Fats**: Choose items low in saturated and trans fats. Aim for products with healthy unsaturated fats.

- **Sodium Content**: Opt for low-sodium versions of canned goods, broths, and pre-packaged foods.

4. Buy in Bulk

Whole Grains and Legumes

- **Bulk Bins**: Purchase grains like quinoa, brown rice, and oats from bulk bins to save money and reduce packaging waste.

- **Legumes**: Stock up on dried beans, lentils, and chickpeas for cost-effective, nutrient-dense protein sources.

Nuts and Seeds

- **Long Shelf Life**: Buy nuts and seeds in bulk to save money and ensure you always have these healthy snacks on hand.

5. Choose Organic When Possible

Dirty Dozen

- **Prioritize Organic**: For the most pesticide-laden produce like strawberries, spinach, and apples, choose organic to reduce exposure to harmful chemicals.

Clean Fifteen

- **Conventional Options**: For produce with lower pesticide residues like avocados, sweet corn, and pineapples, buying conventional is generally safe.

6. Seasonal and Local Produce

Seasonal Buying

- **Better Quality and Price**: Seasonal fruits and vegetables are often fresher, more nutritious, and cheaper.

- **Variety**: Incorporate seasonal produce to add variety to your diet.

Farmers Markets

- **Local and Fresh**: Support local farmers and get the freshest produce by shopping at farmers markets.

- **Organic Options**: Many local farms use organic practices even if they are not certified organic.

7. Mindful Budgeting

Sales and Discounts

- **Weekly Flyers**: Check store flyers for deals on healthy staples like fresh produce, lean proteins, and whole grains.

- **Coupons**: Use coupons for savings on essential items, but avoid buying unhealthy foods just because they are on sale.

Store Brands

- **Cost-Effective**: Store brands often offer the same quality as name brands at a lower price.

- **Healthy Alternatives**: Look for store-brand versions of healthy staples.

8. Smart Substitutes

Healthier Options

- **Whole Grains**: Substitute white rice with brown rice or quinoa for added nutrients.

- **Plant-Based Milks**: Replace cow's milk with almond, soy, or oat milk for a dairy-free option.

Low-Sodium and Low-Sugar

- **Seasonings**: Use herbs and spices instead of salt to flavor your dishes.

- **Natural Sweeteners**: Choose honey or maple syrup in moderation instead of refined sugars.

By following these tips, you can make your grocery shopping trips more efficient, health-focused, and enjoyable. Stocking your kitchen with the right ingredients ensures that you are always prepared to create delicious and nutritious anti-inflammatory meals, supporting your overall wellness and lifestyle goals.

BREAKFAST IDEAS

Berry Spinach Smoothie Bowl

Servings: 2

Cooking Time:

- **Prep Time:** 10 minutes
- **Cook Time:** N/A
- **Total Time:** 10 minutes

Ingredients:

- 1 cup spinach leaves
- 1 cup mixed berries (strawberries, blueberries, raspberries)
- 1 banana
- 1/2 cup almond milk (or any plant-based milk)
- 1 tbsp chia seeds
- 1 tbsp almond butter
- 1 tbsp honey or maple syrup (optional)

Toppings:

- Sliced banana
- Fresh berries
- Granola
- Coconut flakes

Instructions:

1. In a blender, combine spinach, mixed berries, banana, almond milk, chia seeds, almond butter, and honey or maple syrup (if using).
2. Blend until smooth and creamy.
3. Pour the smoothie into bowls.
4. Top with sliced banana, fresh berries, granola, and coconut flakes.
5. Serve immediately and enjoy!

Nutritional Information (approximate): Calories per serving: 300; Protein: 6g; Fat: 10g; Saturated Fat: 2g; Carbohydrates: 45g; Fiber: 9g; Sugar: 22g; Sodium: 100mg

Tips and Variations:

- Use frozen berries for a thicker consistency.
- Add a scoop of protein powder for extra protein.
- Substitute almond butter with peanut butter or sunflower seed butter.

Servings: 2

Cooking Time:

- **Prep Time:** 5 minutes
- **Cook Time:** N/A
- **Total Time:** 5 minutes + overnight soaking

Ingredients:

- 1 cup rolled oats
- 1 cup almond milk (or any plant-based milk)
- 1/2 cup blueberries
- 2 tbsp chia seeds
- 1 tbsp honey or maple syrup
- 1/2 tsp vanilla extract

Toppings:

- Fresh blueberries
- Sliced almonds
- Coconut flakes

Instructions:

1. In a jar or container, combine rolled oats, almond milk, blueberries, chia seeds, honey or maple syrup, and vanilla extract.
2. Stir well to combine.
3. Cover and refrigerate overnight or for at least 4 hours.

4. In the morning, stir the oats and add a bit more almond milk if needed to reach desired consistency.

5. Top with fresh blueberries, sliced almonds, and coconut flakes.

6. Serve and enjoy!

Nutritional Information (approximate): Calories per serving: 350; Protein: 10g; Fat: 10g; Saturated Fat: 2g; Carbohydrates: 55g; Fiber: 12g; Sugar: 12g; Sodium: 100mg

Tips and Variations:

- Use any type of fruit instead of blueberries, such as strawberries, raspberries, or diced mango.
- Add a spoonful of nut butter for extra creaminess and protein.
- Substitute rolled oats with steel-cut oats for a different texture.

Servings: 2

Cooking Time:

- **Prep Time:** 10 minutes
- **Cook Time:** N/A
- **Total Time:** 10 minutes

Ingredients:

- 1 banana
- 1 cup pineapple chunks
- 1 cup coconut water
- 1/2 tsp ground turmeric
- 1/2-inch fresh ginger, peeled and grated
- 1 tbsp chia seeds
- 1 tbsp honey or maple syrup (optional)

Instructions:

1. In a blender, combine banana, pineapple chunks, coconut water, ground turmeric, grated ginger, chia seeds, and honey or maple syrup (if using).
2. Blend until smooth and creamy.
3. Pour into glasses and serve immediately.
4. Enjoy!

Nutritional Information (approximate): Calories per serving: 180; Protein: 2g; Fat: 3g; Saturated Fat: 1g; Carbohydrates: 40g; Fiber: 5g; Sugar: 25g; Sodium: 45mg

Tips and Variations:

- Use fresh turmeric if available; a small piece of peeled turmeric root works well.
- Add a handful of spinach for an extra nutrient boost.
- Adjust the sweetness by adding more or less honey or maple syrup.

Servings: 2

Cooking Time:

- **Prep Time:** 5 minutes
- **Cook Time:** 20 minutes
- **Total Time:** 25 minutes

Ingredients:

- 1 cup cooked quinoa
- 1 cup almond milk (or any plant-based milk)
- 1 tbsp honey or maple syrup
- 1/2 tsp cinnamon
- 1/4 tsp vanilla extract
- Fresh fruit (such as berries, banana slices, or diced apple)
- Nuts and seeds (such as almonds, walnuts, or chia seeds)

Instructions:

1. In a saucepan, combine cooked quinoa, almond milk, honey or maple syrup, cinnamon, and vanilla extract.
2. Bring to a simmer over medium heat, stirring occasionally.
3. Cook for 5-7 minutes, until the mixture thickens and is heated through.
4. Divide the porridge into bowls.
5. Top with fresh fruit, nuts, and seeds.
6. Serve warm and enjoy!

Nutritional Information (approximate): Calories per serving: 250; Protein: 8g; Fat: 7g; Saturated Fat: 1g; Carbohydrates: 40g; Fiber: 5g; Sugar: 12g; Sodium: 75mg

Tips and Variations:

- Use leftover quinoa or prepare it in advance to save time.
- Add a spoonful of nut butter for extra protein and creaminess.
- Experiment with different spices like nutmeg or cardamom for a unique flavor.

Servings: 2

Cooking Time:

- **Prep Time:** 10 minutes
- **Cook Time:** N/A
- **Total Time:** 10 minutes + overnight chilling

Ingredients:

- 1/2 cup chia seeds
- 2 cups coconut milk (or any plant-based milk)
- 1 tbsp honey or maple syrup
- 1 tsp vanilla extract
- 1 ripe mango, diced
- 1/4 cup shredded coconut

Instructions:

1. In a bowl, combine chia seeds, coconut milk, honey or maple syrup, and vanilla extract.
2. Stir well to combine and let sit for 5 minutes.
3. Stir again to prevent clumping, then cover and refrigerate overnight or for at least 4 hours.
4. When ready to serve, divide the chia pudding into bowls.
5. Top with diced mango and shredded coconut.
6. Serve and enjoy!

Nutritional Information (approximate): Calories per serving: 300; Protein: 6g; Fat: 20g; Saturated Fat: 15g; Carbohydrates: 25g; Fiber: 10g; Sugar: 15g; Sodium: 25mg

Tips and Variations:
- Use any type of fruit instead of mango, such as berries, kiwi, or pineapple.
- Add a sprinkle of nuts or seeds for extra texture and nutrition.
- Use light coconut milk for a lower-fat option.

Servings: 2

Cooking Time:

- **Prep Time:** 10 minutes
- **Cook Time:** N/A
- **Total Time:** 10 minutes

Ingredients:

- 1 cup kale leaves, stems removed
- 1 cup spinach leaves
- 1 green apple, cored and chopped
- 1 banana
- 1/2 cucumber, chopped
- 1/2 lemon, juiced
- 1 tbsp chia seeds
- 1 cup coconut water (or any plant-based milk)
- 1 tsp fresh ginger, grated (optional)

Instructions:

1. In a blender, combine kale, spinach, green apple, banana, cucumber, lemon juice, chia seeds, coconut water, and fresh ginger (if using).
2. Blend until smooth and creamy.
3. Pour into glasses and serve immediately.
4. Enjoy!

Nutritional Information (approximate): Calories per serving: 150; Protein: 3g; Fat: 3g; Saturated Fat: 1g; Carbohydrates: 33g; Fiber: 7g; Sugar: 18g; Sodium: 35mg

Tips and Variations:

- Add a handful of fresh mint or parsley for extra freshness.
- Use frozen banana for a thicker, creamier texture.
- Adjust the amount of liquid to achieve your desired consistency.

Servings: 2

Cooking Time:

- **Prep Time:** 5 minutes
- **Cook Time:** 10 minutes
- **Total Time:** 15 minutes

Ingredients:

- 1 cup rolled oats
- 2 cups water or almond milk (or any plant-based milk)
- 1 tbsp flaxseeds
- 1 tbsp honey or maple syrup
- 1/2 tsp cinnamon
- 1 cup mixed berries (blueberries, strawberries, raspberries)

Toppings:

- Additional berries
- Nuts and seeds (such as almonds, walnuts, chia seeds)
- A drizzle of honey or maple syrup

Instructions:

1. In a saucepan, bring water or almond milk to a boil.
2. Stir in rolled oats, flaxseeds, honey or maple syrup, and cinnamon.
3. Reduce heat to low and simmer for about 5-7 minutes, stirring occasionally, until the oats are tender and the mixture is creamy.

4. Stir in mixed berries and cook for another 2 minutes.

5. Divide the oatmeal into bowls and top with additional berries, nuts, and seeds.

6. Serve warm and enjoy!

Nutritional Information (approximate): Calories per serving: 300; Protein: 8g; Fat: 8g; Saturated Fat: 1g; Carbohydrates: 50g; Fiber: 10g; Sugar: 12g; Sodium: 50mg

Tips and Variations:

- Use steel-cut oats for a heartier texture; adjust cooking time accordingly.
- Substitute flaxseeds with chia seeds or hemp seeds.
- Add a dollop of nut butter for extra creaminess and protein.

Servings: 2

Cooking Time:

- **Prep Time:** 10 minutes
- **Cook Time:** N/A
- **Total Time:** 10 minutes

Ingredients:

- 2 slices whole-grain bread, toasted
- 1 ripe avocado
- 1/2 cup cherry tomatoes, halved
- Fresh basil leaves, torn
- Salt and pepper, to taste
- A drizzle of olive oil (optional)
- A squeeze of lemon juice (optional)

Instructions:

1. In a small bowl, mash the avocado with a fork until smooth.
2. Spread the mashed avocado evenly over the toasted bread slices.
3. Top with halved cherry tomatoes and torn basil leaves.
4. Season with salt and pepper to taste.
5. Drizzle with olive oil and squeeze lemon juice over the top, if desired.
6. Serve immediately and enjoy!

Nutritional Information (approximate): Calories per serving: 250; Protein: 6g; Fat: 18g; Saturated Fat: 3g; Carbohydrates: 20g; Fiber: 7g; Sugar: 3g; Sodium: 150mg

Tips and Variations:

- Add a poached egg on top for extra protein.
- Use different types of bread, such as sourdough or rye.
- Add red pepper flakes for a spicy kick.

Servings: 2

Cooking Time:

- **Prep Time:** 10 minutes
- **Cook Time:** 20 minutes
- **Total Time:** 30 minutes

Ingredients:

- 2 medium sweet potatoes, peeled and diced
- 1 tbsp olive oil
- 1/2 onion, diced
- 1 red bell pepper, diced
- 2 cups fresh spinach leaves
- 4 eggs
- Salt and pepper, to taste
- Fresh parsley, chopped (optional)

Instructions:

1. In a large skillet, heat olive oil over medium heat.
2. Add diced sweet potatoes and cook for about 10 minutes, stirring occasionally, until they begin to soften.
3. Add diced onion and bell pepper to the skillet and cook for another 5 minutes, until vegetables are tender.
4. Stir in spinach leaves and cook until wilted, about 2 minutes.
5. Create four small wells in the hash mixture and crack an egg into each well.

6. Cover the skillet and cook for about 5 minutes, or until eggs are cooked to your liking.

7. Season with salt and pepper, and sprinkle with chopped parsley, if desired.

8. Serve hot and enjoy!

Nutritional Information (approximate): Calories per serving: 350; Protein: 14g; Fat: 18g; Saturated Fat: 4g; Carbohydrates: 35g; Fiber: 8g; Sugar: 10g; Sodium: 200mg

Tips and Variations:

- Add cooked sausage or bacon for a non-vegetarian option.
- Substitute spinach with kale or Swiss chard.
- Top with hot sauce or salsa for extra flavor.

Servings: 12 muffins

Cooking Time:

- **Prep Time:** 15 minutes
- **Cook Time:** 25 minutes
- **Total Time:** 40 minutes

Ingredients:

- 10 large eggs
- 1/2 cup almond milk (or any plant-based milk)
- 1 cup spinach, chopped
- 1 cup mushrooms, diced
- 1/2 cup bell pepper, diced
- 1/4 cup green onions, chopped
- Salt and pepper, to taste
- 1/2 cup shredded cheese (optional)

Instructions:

1. Preheat oven to 375°F (190°C).
2. Grease a 12-cup muffin tin or line with muffin liners.
3. In a large bowl, whisk together eggs and almond milk.
4. Stir in chopped spinach, mushrooms, bell pepper, green onions, salt, and pepper.
5. Pour the egg mixture evenly into the muffin cups.
6. Sprinkle shredded cheese on top, if using.

7. Bake for 20-25 minutes, or until the muffins are set and lightly golden.

8. Let cool slightly before removing from the muffin tin.

9. Serve warm or store in the refrigerator for up to 5 days.

Nutritional Information (approximate): Calories per muffin: 80; Protein: 7g; Fat: 5g; Saturated Fat: 1.5g; Carbohydrates: 2g; Fiber: 0.5g; Sugar: 1g; Sodium: 120mg

Tips and Variations:
- Add cooked bacon or sausage for extra protein.
- Substitute other vegetables such as zucchini, broccoli, or tomatoes.
- Freeze extra muffins for a quick and easy breakfast option.

Servings: 2

Cooking Time:

- **Prep Time:** 5 minutes
- **Cook Time:** N/A
- **Total Time:** 5 minutes

Ingredients:

- 2 slices whole-grain bread, toasted
- 2 tbsp almond butter
- 1 banana, sliced
- A sprinkle of cinnamon
- A drizzle of honey (optional)

Instructions:

1. Spread almond butter evenly over the toasted bread slices.
2. Top with banana slices.
3. Sprinkle with cinnamon and drizzle with honey, if desired.
4. Serve immediately and enjoy!

Nutritional Information (approximate): Calories per serving: 250; Protein: 6g; Fat: 12g; Saturated Fat: 1g; Carbohydrates: 30g; Fiber: 5g; Sugar: 12g; Sodium: 150mg

Tips and Variations:

- Use peanut butter or cashew butter instead of almond butter.
- Add chia seeds or flaxseeds for extra nutrition.
- Top with fresh berries or a sprinkle of granola.

Servings: 2

Cooking Time:

- **Prep Time:** 10 minutes
- **Cook Time:** N/A
- **Total Time:** 10 minutes

Ingredients:

- 1 cup pumpkin puree
- 1 banana
- 1 cup almond milk (or any plant-based milk)
- 1/2 cup Greek yogurt (or dairy-free yogurt)
- 1 tbsp honey or maple syrup
- 1/2 tsp pumpkin pie spice
- 1/2 tsp cinnamon
- 1 tsp vanilla extract
- Ice cubes (optional)

Instructions:

1. In a blender, combine pumpkin puree, banana, almond milk, Greek yogurt, honey or maple syrup, pumpkin pie spice, cinnamon, vanilla extract, and ice cubes (if using).
2. Blend until smooth and creamy.
3. Pour into glasses and serve immediately.
4. Enjoy!

Nutritional Information (approximate): Calories per serving: 180; Protein: 6g; Fat: 2g; Saturated Fat: 0.5g; Carbohydrates: 36g; Fiber: 5g; Sugar: 18g; Sodium: 90mg

Tips and Variations:

- Add a scoop of protein powder for extra protein.
- Use frozen banana for a thicker, creamier texture.
- Adjust the sweetness by adding more or less honey or maple syrup.

Servings: 12 (1/2 cup per serving)

Cooking Time:

- **Prep Time:** 10 minutes
- **Cook Time:** 25 minutes
- **Total Time:** 35 minutes

Ingredients:

- 3 cups rolled oats
- 1 cup shredded coconut
- 1 cup sliced almonds
- 1/4 cup chia seeds
- 1/4 cup coconut oil, melted
- 1/4 cup honey or maple syrup
- 1 tsp vanilla extract
- 1/2 tsp cinnamon
- 1/4 tsp salt

Instructions:

1. Preheat oven to 325°F (160°C).
2. In a large bowl, combine rolled oats, shredded coconut, sliced almonds, and chia seeds.
3. In a small bowl, whisk together melted coconut oil, honey or maple syrup, vanilla extract, cinnamon, and salt.
4. Pour the wet ingredients over the dry ingredients and stir to combine.

5. Spread the mixture evenly on a baking sheet lined with parchment paper.

6. Bake for 20-25 minutes, stirring halfway through, until golden brown.

7. Let cool completely before storing in an airtight container.

8. Serve with yogurt, milk, or as a snack.

Nutritional Information (approximate): Calories per serving: 250; Protein: 5g; Fat: 15g; Saturated Fat: 8g; Carbohydrates: 25g; Fiber: 5g; Sugar: 8g; Sodium: 75mg

Tips and Variations:

- Add dried fruit such as cranberries, raisins, or chopped apricots after baking.
- Substitute sliced almonds with other nuts like walnuts, pecans, or cashews.
- Add a sprinkle of cacao nibs or dark chocolate chips for a treat.

LUNCH AND DINNER RECIPES

Grilled Salmon with Quinoa and Asparagus

Servings: 4

Cooking Time:

- **Prep Time:** 15 minutes
- **Cook Time:** 20 minutes
- **Total Time:** 35 minutes

Ingredients:

- 4 salmon fillets
- 1 cup quinoa, rinsed
- 2 cups vegetable broth
- 1 bunch asparagus, trimmed
- 2 tbsp olive oil
- 1 lemon, sliced
- 2 cloves garlic, minced
- Salt and pepper, to taste
- Fresh dill or parsley, for garnish

Instructions:

1. Preheat grill to medium-high heat.
2. In a medium saucepan, bring vegetable broth to a boil. Add quinoa, reduce heat to low, cover, and simmer for 15 minutes or until liquid is absorbed. Fluff with a fork.

3. While quinoa is cooking, toss asparagus with 1 tbsp olive oil, minced garlic, salt, and pepper.

4. Grill salmon fillets and asparagus for about 4-5 minutes per side, until salmon is cooked through and asparagus is tender.

5. Serve salmon over quinoa, with grilled asparagus on the side. Garnish with lemon slices and fresh dill or parsley.

6. Enjoy!

Nutritional Information (approximate): Calories per serving: 400; Protein: 30g; Fat: 20g; Saturated Fat: 3g; Carbohydrates: 25g; Fiber: 5g; Sugar: 2g; Sodium: 350mg

Tips and Variations:
- Add a sprinkle of red pepper flakes for a spicy kick.
- Substitute salmon with another fish such as trout or cod.
- Use mixed vegetables instead of just asparagus for more variety.

Servings: 6

Cooking Time:

- **Prep Time:** 15 minutes
- **Cook Time:** 40 minutes
- **Total Time:** 55 minutes

Ingredients:

- 1 cup green or brown lentils, rinsed
- 1 tbsp olive oil
- 1 onion, diced
- 3 cloves garlic, minced
- 2 carrots, diced
- 2 celery stalks, diced
- 1 bell pepper, diced
- 1 zucchini, diced
- 1 can diced tomatoes
- 4 cups vegetable broth
- 1 tsp ground cumin
- 1 tsp smoked paprika
- 1 bay leaf
- Salt and pepper, to taste
- Fresh parsley, chopped (optional)

Instructions:

1. In a large pot, heat olive oil over medium heat. Add onion and garlic, and sauté until translucent, about 5 minutes.
2. Add carrots, celery, bell pepper, and zucchini. Cook for another 5 minutes, stirring occasionally.
3. Stir in lentils, diced tomatoes, vegetable broth, cumin, smoked paprika, bay leaf, salt, and pepper.
4. Bring to a boil, then reduce heat and simmer for 30-35 minutes, or until lentils and vegetables are tender.
5. Remove bay leaf, adjust seasoning if necessary, and serve hot, garnished with fresh parsley.
6. Enjoy!

Nutritional Information (approximate): Calories per serving: 250; Protein: 12g; Fat: 5g; Saturated Fat: 1g; Carbohydrates: 40g; Fiber: 15g; Sugar: 10g; Sodium: 500mg

Tips and Variations:

- Add a handful of spinach or kale at the end of cooking for extra greens.
- Use red lentils for a quicker cooking time.
- Add a dash of hot sauce or chili flakes for extra heat.

Servings: 4

Cooking Time:
- **Prep Time:** 10 minutes
- **Cook Time:** 30 minutes
- **Total Time:** 40 minutes

Ingredients:
- 1 head cauliflower, cut into florets
- 1 can chickpeas, drained and rinsed
- 2 tbsp olive oil
- 1 tsp ground turmeric
- 1 tsp ground cumin
- 1/2 tsp paprika
- Salt and pepper, to taste
- 1/4 cup fresh parsley, chopped
- 1 lemon, cut into wedges

Instructions:
1. Preheat oven to 400°F (200°C).
2. In a large bowl, toss cauliflower florets and chickpeas with olive oil, turmeric, cumin, paprika, salt, and pepper until evenly coated.
3. Spread the mixture on a baking sheet in a single layer.
4. Roast in the preheated oven for 25-30 minutes, or until cauliflower is tender and lightly browned, stirring halfway through.

5. Remove from oven and sprinkle with fresh parsley.

6. Serve with lemon wedges on the side.

7. Enjoy!

Nutritional Information (approximate): Calories per serving: 200; Protein: 6g; Fat: 10g; Saturated Fat: 1.5g; Carbohydrates: 24g; Fiber: 8g; Sugar: 5g; Sodium: 400mg

Tips and Variations:

- Serve over quinoa or brown rice for a more filling meal.
- Add other vegetables like carrots or bell peppers for more variety.
- Top with a dollop of plain yogurt or tahini sauce for extra creaminess.

Servings: 4

Cooking Time:

- **Prep Time:** 15 minutes
- **Cook Time:** 30 minutes
- **Total Time:** 45 minutes

Ingredients:

- 1 medium butternut squash, peeled and diced
- 2 tbsp olive oil
- Salt and pepper, to taste
- 1 bunch kale, stems removed and chopped
- 1/4 cup dried cranberries
- 1/4 cup pumpkin seeds
- 1/4 cup crumbled feta cheese (optional)

Dressing:

- 1/4 cup olive oil
- 2 tbsp apple cider vinegar
- 1 tbsp maple syrup
- 1 tsp Dijon mustard
- Salt and pepper, to taste

Instructions:

1. Preheat oven to 400°F (200°C).
2. Toss butternut squash with 2 tbsp olive oil, salt, and pepper. Spread on a baking sheet and roast for 25-30 minutes, or until tender and lightly browned.
3. While squash is roasting, massage chopped kale with a pinch of salt for about 2 minutes to soften.
4. In a small bowl, whisk together the dressing ingredients: olive oil, apple cider vinegar, maple syrup, Dijon mustard, salt, and pepper.
5. In a large bowl, combine roasted butternut squash, massaged kale, dried cranberries, pumpkin seeds, and crumbled feta (if using).
6. Drizzle with dressing and toss to combine.
7. Serve immediately and enjoy!

Nutritional Information (approximate): Calories per serving: 250; Protein: 5g; Fat: 18g; Saturated Fat: 3g; Carbohydrates: 20g; Fiber: 5g; Sugar: 8g; Sodium: 300mg

Tips and Variations:

- Add cooked quinoa for extra protein and texture.
- Use spinach or arugula instead of kale.
- Top with grilled chicken or tofu for a more substantial meal.

Servings: 4

Cooking Time:

- **Prep Time:** 15 minutes
- **Cook Time:** 5 minutes
- **Total Time:** 20 minutes

Ingredients:

- 4 medium zucchinis, spiralized
- 1 cup cherry tomatoes, halved
- 1/2 cup basil pesto (store-bought or homemade)
- 1/4 cup pine nuts, toasted
- Salt and pepper, to taste
- Fresh basil leaves, for garnish

Instructions:

1. In a large bowl, toss zucchini noodles with cherry tomatoes and pesto until well combined.
2. Heat a large skillet over medium heat. Add the zucchini noodle mixture and cook for 2-3 minutes, until just tender.
3. Season with salt and pepper to taste.
4. Transfer to serving bowls and top with toasted pine nuts and fresh basil leaves.
5. Serve immediately and enjoy!

Nutritional Information (approximate): Calories per serving: 200; Protein: 4g; Fat: 18g; Saturated Fat: 2.5g; Carbohydrates: 10g; Fiber: 3g; Sugar: 5g; Sodium: 250mg

Tips and Variations:

- Add grilled chicken or shrimp for extra protein.
- Use a different type of pesto, such as sun-dried tomato or arugula pesto.
- Substitute zucchini noodles with spaghetti squash or butternut squash noodles.

Servings: 4

Cooking Time:

- **Prep Time:** 10 minutes
- **Cook Time:** 20 minutes
- **Total Time:** 30 minutes

Ingredients:

- 1 cup quinoa, rinsed
- 2 cups vegetable broth
- 1 tbsp olive oil
- 1 onion, diced
- 3 cloves garlic, minced
- 2 cups mushrooms, sliced
- 4 cups fresh spinach, chopped
- Salt and pepper, to taste
- Fresh parsley, chopped (optional)

Instructions:

1. In a medium saucepan, bring vegetable broth to a boil. Add quinoa, reduce heat to low, cover, and simmer for 15 minutes or until liquid is absorbed. Fluff with a fork.

2. In a large skillet, heat olive oil over medium heat. Add onion and garlic, and sauté until translucent, about 5 minutes.

3. Add mushrooms and cook until they release their moisture and become tender, about 5-7 minutes.

4. Stir in chopped spinach and cook until wilted, about 2 minutes.

5. Add cooked quinoa to the skillet and stir to combine. Season with salt and pepper to taste.

6. Serve hot, garnished with fresh parsley if desired.

7. Enjoy!

Nutritional Information (approximate): Calories per serving: 250; Protein: 8g; Fat: 8g; Saturated Fat: 1g; Carbohydrates: 35g; Fiber: 6g; Sugar: 4g; Sodium: 400mg

Tips and Variations:
- Add a sprinkle of nutritional yeast for a cheesy flavor.
- Use kale or Swiss chard instead of spinach.
- Top with a poached egg for extra protein.

Servings: 4

Cooking Time:

- **Prep Time:** 15 minutes
- **Cook Time:** 10 minutes
- **Total Time:** 25 minutes

Ingredients:

- 1 lb ground chicken
- 1 tbsp olive oil
- 1 onion, diced
- 2 cloves garlic, minced
- 1 red bell pepper, diced
- 2 carrots, shredded
- 1/4 cup soy sauce or tamari
- 2 tbsp hoisin sauce
- 1 tbsp rice vinegar
- 1 tsp sriracha (optional)
- 1 head butter lettuce, leaves separated
- 1/4 cup chopped peanuts
- Fresh cilantro, chopped

Instructions:

1. In a large skillet, heat olive oil over medium heat. Add onion and garlic, and sauté until translucent, about 5 minutes.

2. Add ground chicken and cook until no longer pink, breaking it up with a wooden spoon.
3. Stir in bell pepper, carrots, soy sauce, hoisin sauce, rice vinegar, and sriracha (if using). Cook for another 5 minutes, until vegetables are tender and sauce has thickened.
4. Remove from heat and spoon the mixture into lettuce leaves.
5. Top with chopped peanuts and fresh cilantro.
6. Serve immediately and enjoy!

Nutritional Information (approximate): Calories per serving: 300; Protein: 25g; Fat: 15g; Saturated Fat: 3g; Carbohydrates: 15g; Fiber: 4g; Sugar: 5g; Sodium: 700mg

Tips and Variations:
- Use ground turkey or beef instead of chicken.
- Add water chestnuts or mushrooms for extra crunch.
- Serve with a side of jasmine rice for a more filling meal.

Servings: 4

Cooking Time:

- **Prep Time:** 10 minutes
- **Cook Time:** 10 minutes
- **Total Time:** 20 minutes

Ingredients:

- 1 lb large shrimp, peeled and deveined
- 2 tbsp olive oil
- 4 cloves garlic, minced
- 1/4 cup lemon juice
- 1/4 cup vegetable broth
- 4 medium zucchinis, spiralized
- Salt and pepper, to taste
- Fresh parsley, chopped

Instructions:

1. In a large skillet, heat olive oil over medium-high heat. Add garlic and sauté for 1 minute, until fragrant.
2. Add shrimp and cook for 2-3 minutes on each side, until pink and opaque.
3. Stir in lemon juice and vegetable broth. Cook for another 2 minutes, until sauce is slightly reduced.
4. Add spiralized zucchini noodles (zoodles) to the skillet and toss to combine. Cook for 2-3 minutes, until zoodles are tender.
5. Season with salt and pepper to taste.

6. Serve hot, garnished with fresh parsley.

7. Enjoy!

Nutritional Information (approximate): Calories per serving: 250; Protein: 25g; Fat: 10g; Saturated Fat: 1.5g; Carbohydrates: 15g; Fiber: 4g; Sugar: 6g; Sodium: 600mg

Tips and Variations:

- Add cherry tomatoes or bell peppers for extra color and flavor.
- Use a different type of pasta, such as spaghetti squash or shirataki noodles.
- Top with grated Parmesan cheese for a cheesy finish.

Servings: 4

Cooking Time:
- **Prep Time:** 15 minutes
- **Cook Time:** 20 minutes
- **Total Time:** 35 minutes

Ingredients:
- 4 large portobello mushrooms, stems removed
- 1 tbsp olive oil
- 1 onion, diced
- 3 cloves garlic, minced
- 1 red bell pepper, diced
- 1 zucchini, diced
- 1 cup spinach, chopped
- 1/4 cup breadcrumbs (gluten-free if needed)
- 1/4 cup grated Parmesan cheese (optional)
- Salt and pepper, to taste
- Fresh parsley, chopped (optional)

Instructions:
1. Preheat oven to 375°F (190°C).
2. In a large skillet, heat olive oil over medium heat. Add onion and garlic, and sauté until translucent, about 5 minutes.
3. Add bell pepper and zucchini, and cook until tender, about 5 minutes.

4. Stir in chopped spinach and cook until wilted, about 2 minutes.

5. Remove from heat and stir in breadcrumbs and Parmesan cheese (if using). Season with salt and pepper to taste.

6. Place portobello mushrooms on a baking sheet and spoon the vegetable mixture into each mushroom cap.

7. Bake in the preheated oven for 20 minutes, or until mushrooms are tender.

8. Serve hot, garnished with fresh parsley if desired.

9. Enjoy!

Nutritional Information (approximate): Calories per serving: 200; Protein: 6g; Fat: 10g; Saturated Fat: 2g; Carbohydrates: 25g; Fiber: 5g; Sugar: 8g; Sodium: 400mg

Tips and Variations:

- Add cooked quinoa or rice to the stuffing mixture for extra bulk.
- Use different vegetables like cherry tomatoes or eggplant.
- Top with a slice of mozzarella cheese before baking for a cheesy finish.

Servings: 4

Cooking Time:

- **Prep Time:** 15 minutes
- **Cook Time:** 15 minutes
- **Total Time:** 30 minutes

Ingredients:

- 1 lb. boneless, skinless chicken breasts, thinly sliced
- 2 tbsp olive oil
- 1 onion, sliced
- 3 cloves garlic, minced
- 1 red bell pepper, sliced
- 1 yellow bell pepper, sliced
- 2 cups broccoli florets
- 2 carrots, julienned
- 1/4 cup soy sauce or tamari
- 2 tbsp hoisin sauce
- 1 tbsp rice vinegar
- 1 tsp sesame oil
- 1 tsp grated ginger
- Salt and pepper, to taste
- Sesame seeds, for garnish
- Fresh cilantro, chopped

Instructions:

1. In a large skillet or wok, heat 1 tbsp olive oil over medium-high heat. Add chicken and cook until browned and cooked through, about 5-7 minutes. Remove from skillet and set aside.

2. In the same skillet, add remaining 1 tbsp olive oil. Add onion and garlic, and sauté until translucent, about 5 minutes.

3. Add bell peppers, broccoli, and carrots. Cook until vegetables are tender-crisp, about 5-7 minutes.

4. In a small bowl, whisk together soy sauce, hoisin sauce, rice vinegar, sesame oil, and grated ginger.

5. Return chicken to the skillet and pour sauce over the mixture. Stir to combine and cook for another 2-3 minutes, until everything is heated through and sauce has thickened slightly.

6. Season with salt and pepper to taste.

7. Serve hot, garnished with sesame seeds and fresh cilantro.

8. Enjoy!

Nutritional Information (approximate): Calories per serving: 350; Protein: 30g; Fat: 15g; Saturated Fat: 2.5g; Carbohydrates: 20g; Fiber: 5g; Sugar: 10g; Sodium: 800mg

Tips and Variations:

- Serve over brown rice, quinoa, or cauliflower rice for a complete meal.
- Substitute chicken with beef, shrimp, or tofu.
- Add snow peas, snap peas, or baby corn for more variety.

Servings: 4

Cooking Time:

- **Prep Time:** 10 minutes
- **Cook Time:** 30 minutes
- **Total Time:** 40 minutes

Ingredients:

- 4 cod fillets
- 2 large sweet potatoes, peeled and diced
- 2 cups Brussels sprouts, halved
- 3 tbsp olive oil
- 1 lemon, sliced
- 2 cloves garlic, minced
- 1 tsp smoked paprika
- Salt and pepper, to taste
- Fresh parsley, chopped (optional)

Instructions:

1. Preheat oven to 400°F (200°C).
2. In a large bowl, toss diced sweet potatoes and Brussels sprouts with 2 tbsp olive oil, minced garlic, smoked paprika, salt, and pepper.
3. Spread the vegetables on a baking sheet in a single layer and roast for 20 minutes.

4. Remove from oven and place cod fillets on the same baking sheet. Drizzle with remaining 1 tbsp olive oil, and season with salt and pepper. Add lemon slices on top of the cod.
5. Return to oven and bake for an additional 10-12 minutes, or until cod is cooked through and flakes easily with a fork.
6. Serve hot, garnished with fresh parsley if desired.
7. Enjoy!

Nutritional Information (approximate): Calories per serving: 350; Protein: 30g; Fat: 12g; Saturated Fat: 2g; Carbohydrates: 35g; Fiber: 8g; Sugar: 10g; Sodium: 400mg

Tips and Variations:
- Substitute cod with another white fishes like haddock or halibut.
- Add a drizzle of balsamic glaze over the roasted vegetables for extra flavor.
- Serve with a side of steamed rice or quinoa for a more filling meal.

Servings: 4

Cooking Time:

- **Prep Time:** 15 minutes
- **Cook Time:** 0 minutes
- **Total Time:** 15 minutes

Ingredients:

- 1 can chickpeas, drained and rinsed
- 1 cucumber, diced
- 1 cup cherry tomatoes, halved
- 1/2 red onion, thinly sliced
- 1/4 cup Kalamata olives, pitted and halved
- 1/4 cup feta cheese, crumbled (optional)
- 1/4 cup fresh parsley, chopped

Dressing:

- 1/4 cup olive oil
- 2 tbsp red wine vinegar
- 1 tsp dried oregano
- Salt and pepper, to taste

Instructions:

1. In a large bowl, combine chickpeas, cucumber, cherry tomatoes, red onion, Kalamata olives, feta cheese (if using), and fresh parsley.

2. In a small bowl, whisk together olive oil, red wine vinegar, dried oregano, salt, and pepper.

3. Pour dressing over the salad and toss to combine.

4. Serve immediately or refrigerate for up to 2 days.

5. Enjoy!

Nutritional Information (approximate): Calories per serving: 250; Protein: 8g; Fat: 16g; Saturated Fat: 3g; Carbohydrates: 20g; Fiber: 6g; Sugar: 4g; Sodium: 500mg

Tips and Variations:

- Add diced avocado for extra creaminess.
- Use lemon juice instead of red wine vinegar for a different flavor.
- Serve over a bed of mixed greens for a more substantial salad.

Servings: 4

Cooking Time:

- **Prep Time:** 15 minutes
- **Cook Time:** 20 minutes
- **Total Time:** 35 minutes

Ingredients:

- 1 cup quinoa, rinsed
- 2 cups vegetable broth
- 1 tbsp olive oil
- 1 onion, diced
- 3 cloves garlic, minced
- 1 can black beans, drained and rinsed
- 1 tsp ground cumin
- 1 tsp chili powder
- Salt and pepper, to taste
- 8 small corn tortillas
- 1 cup shredded lettuce
- 1/2 cup diced tomatoes
- 1/4 cup chopped cilantro
- 1 avocado, sliced
- Lime wedges, for serving

Instructions:

1. In a medium saucepan, bring vegetable broth to a boil. Add quinoa, reduce heat to low, cover, and simmer for 15 minutes or until liquid is absorbed. Fluff with a fork.
2. In a large skillet, heat olive oil over medium heat. Add onion and garlic, and sauté until translucent, about 5 minutes.
3. Stir in cooked quinoa, black beans, cumin, chili powder, salt, and pepper. Cook for another 5 minutes, until heated through.
4. Warm tortillas in a dry skillet or microwave.
5. Fill each tortilla with quinoa and black bean mixture. Top with shredded lettuce, diced tomatoes, chopped cilantro, and avocado slices.
6. Serve with lime wedges on the side.
7. Enjoy!

Nutritional Information (approximate): Calories per serving: 350; Protein: 12g; Fat: 15g; Saturated Fat: 2.5g; Carbohydrates: 45g; Fiber: 12g; Sugar: 4g; Sodium: 400mg

Tips and Variations:

- Add a drizzle of hot sauce or salsa for extra flavor.
- Use whole wheat tortillas or lettuce wraps instead of corn tortillas.
- Top with a dollop of Greek yogurt or sour cream for added creaminess.

SNACKS AND APPETIZERS

Guacamole with Veggie Sticks

Servings: 4

Cooking Time:

- **Prep Time:** 10 minutes
- **Cook Time:** 0 minutes
- **Total Time:** 10 minutes

Ingredients:

- 3 ripe avocados
- 1 lime, juiced
- 1/2 cup red onion, finely chopped
- 1 jalapeño, minced (optional)
- 1/4 cup fresh cilantro, chopped
- Salt and pepper, to taste
- Assorted veggie sticks (carrots, celery, bell peppers, cucumbers)

Instructions:

1. In a medium bowl, mash the avocados with a fork until smooth.
2. Stir in lime juice, red onion, jalapeño (if using), cilantro, salt, and pepper.
3. Serve immediately with assorted veggie sticks.
4. Enjoy!

Nutritional Information (approximate): Calories per serving: 220; Protein: 2g; Fat: 20g; Saturated Fat: 3g; Carbohydrates: 12g; Fiber: 9g; Sugar: 2g; Sodium: 150mg

Tips and Variations:

- Add diced tomatoes for extra texture.
- Use lemon juice instead of lime for a different flavor.
- Store in an airtight container with plastic wrap directly on the surface of the guacamole to prevent browning.

Roasted Chickpeas

Servings: 4

Cooking Time:

- **Prep Time:** 10 minutes
- **Cook Time:** 40 minutes
- **Total Time:** 50 minutes

Ingredients:

- 1 can chickpeas, drained and rinsed
- 2 tbsp olive oil
- 1 tsp ground turmeric
- 1/2 tsp ground cumin
- 1/2 tsp paprika

- 1/2 tsp garlic powder
- Salt and pepper, to taste

Instructions:

1. Preheat oven to 400°F (200°C).
2. Pat chickpeas dry with a paper towel. Spread them on a baking sheet.
3. Drizzle with olive oil and sprinkle with turmeric, cumin, paprika, garlic powder, salt, and pepper. Toss to coat evenly.
4. Roast in the oven for 35-40 minutes, stirring halfway through, until chickpeas are golden and crispy.
5. Allow to cool slightly before serving.
6. Enjoy!

Nutritional Information (approximate): Calories per serving: 180; Protein: 6g; Fat: 9g; Saturated Fat: 1.5g; Carbohydrates: 20g; Fiber: 6g; Sugar: 1g; Sodium: 300mg

Tips and Variations:

- Add a squeeze of lemon juice for a zesty finish.
- Store leftovers in an airtight container to maintain crispiness.

Servings: 4

Cooking Time:

- **Prep Time:** 10 minutes
- **Cook Time:** 0 minutes
- **Total Time:** 10 minutes

Ingredients:

- 1 can chickpeas, drained and rinsed
- 1/4 cup tahini
- 2 tbsp olive oil
- 1 lemon, juiced
- 2 cloves garlic, minced
- 1/2 tsp ground cumin
- Salt, to taste
- 1/4 cup water (or as needed for consistency)
- 2 cucumbers, sliced

Instructions:

1. In a food processor, combine chickpeas, tahini, olive oil, lemon juice, garlic, cumin, and salt. Blend until smooth.
2. Add water, a tablespoon at a time, to reach desired consistency.
3. Serve with cucumber slices.
4. Enjoy!

Nutritional Information (approximate): Calories per serving: 200; Protein: 6g; Fat: 12g; Saturated Fat: 1.5g; Carbohydrates: 18g; Fiber: 6g; Sugar: 2g; Sodium: 300mg

Tips and Variations:

- Add roasted red peppers or sun-dried tomatoes to the hummus for extra flavor.
- Use as a spread for sandwiches or wraps.
- Store in the refrigerator for up to 5 days.

Baked Sweet Potato Fries

Servings: 4

Cooking Time:

- **Prep Time:** 10 minutes
- **Cook Time:** 30 minutes
- **Total Time:** 40 minutes

Ingredients:

- 2 large sweet potatoes, cut into fries
- 2 tbsp olive oil
- 1 tsp paprika
- 1/2 tsp garlic powder
- 1/2 tsp salt

- 1/4 tsp black pepper

Instructions:

1. Preheat oven to 425°F (220°C).
2. In a large bowl, toss sweet potato fries with olive oil, paprika, garlic powder, salt, and pepper.
3. Spread fries on a baking sheet in a single layer.
4. Bake for 25-30 minutes, flipping halfway through, until crispy and golden.
5. Serve hot.
6. Enjoy!

Nutritional Information (approximate): Calories per serving: 180; Protein: 2g; Fat: 9g; Saturated Fat: 1.5g; Carbohydrates: 25g; Fiber: 4g; Sugar: 5g; Sodium: 300mg

Tips and Variations:

- Serve with a dipping sauce like guacamole or hummus.
- Sprinkle with fresh herbs like rosemary or thyme before baking.
- Try using different root vegetables like carrots or parsnips.

Servings: 4

Cooking Time:

- **Prep Time:** 5 minutes
- **Cook Time:** 0 minutes
- **Total Time:** 5 minutes

Ingredients:

- 1/2 cup almonds
- 1/2 cup walnuts
- 1/2 cup cashews
- 1/4 cup pumpkin seeds
- 1/4 cup sunflower seeds
- 1/2 cup dried cranberries
- 1/2 cup dried apricots, chopped

Instructions:

1. In a large bowl, combine all ingredients and mix well.
2. Store in an airtight container.
3. Serve as a snack.
4. Enjoy!

Nutritional Information (approximate): Calories per serving: 220; Protein: 6g; Fat: 15g; Saturated Fat: 2g; Carbohydrates: 20g; Fiber: 4g; Sugar: 10g; Sodium: 10mg

Tips and Variations:

- Add dark chocolate chips for a sweet treat.
- Use different nuts and seeds according to preference.
- Perfect for on-the-go snacking or as a topping for yogurt.

Servings: 4

Cooking Time:

- **Prep Time:** 5 minutes
- **Cook Time:** 10 minutes
- **Total Time:** 15 minutes

Ingredients:

- 2 cups edamame in pods
- 1 tbsp sea salt

Instructions:

1. Bring a large pot of water to a boil. Add edamame and cook for 5-7 minutes, until tender.
2. Drain and sprinkle with sea salt.

3. Serve warm.

4. Enjoy!

Nutritional Information (approximate): Calories per serving: 130; Protein: 11g; Fat: 4g; Saturated Fat: 0.5g; Carbohydrates: 10g; Fiber: 4g; Sugar: 1g; Sodium: 300mg

Tips and Variations:

- Add a sprinkle of chili flakes for a spicy kick.
- Serve with a dipping sauce like soy sauce or tamari.

Apple Slices with Almond Butter

Servings: 4

Cooking Time:

- **Prep Time:** 5 minutes
- **Cook Time:** 0 minutes
- **Total Time:** 5 minutes

Ingredients:

- 4 apples, sliced
- 1/2 cup almond butter

Instructions:

1. Slice apples and arrange on a plate.

2. Serve with almond butter for dipping.

3. Enjoy!

Nutritional Information (approximate): Calories per serving: 180; Protein: 4g; Fat: 10g; Saturated Fat: 1g; Carbohydrates: 22g; Fiber: 5g; Sugar: 15g; Sodium: 0mg

Tips and Variations:

- Sprinkle apple slices with cinnamon for extra flavor.
- Use other nut butters like peanut or cashew butter.
- Perfect for a quick and healthy snack.

Greek Yogurt with Berries and Honey

Servings: 4

Cooking Time:

- **Prep Time:** 5 minutes
- **Cook Time:** 0 minutes
- **Total Time:** 5 minutes

Ingredients:

- 2 cups Greek yogurt
- 1 cup mixed berries (strawberries, blueberries, raspberries)
- 2 tbsp honey

Instructions:

1. Divide Greek yogurt into four bowls.
2. Top with mixed berries and drizzle with honey.
3. Serve immediately.
4. Enjoy!

Nutritional Information (approximate): Calories per serving: 150; Protein: 10g; Fat: 4g; Saturated Fat: 2g; Carbohydrates: 20g; Fiber: 2g; Sugar: 15g; Sodium: 50mg

Tips and Variations:

- Add granola for extra crunch.
- Use maple syrup instead of honey.
- Perfect for breakfast or a light snack.

Carrot and Celery Sticks with Tahini Dip

Servings: 4

Cooking Time:

- **Prep Time:** 10 minutes
- **Cook Time:** 0 minutes
- **Total Time:** 10 minutes

Ingredients:

- 4 carrots, cut into sticks
- 4 celery stalks, cut into sticks
- 1/2 cup tahini

- 1 lemon, juiced
- 2 tbsp water (or more, as needed)
- 1 clove garlic, minced
- Salt and pepper, to taste

Instructions:

1. In a small bowl, whisk together tahini, lemon juice, water, garlic, salt, and pepper until smooth.
2. Arrange carrot and celery sticks on a plate.
3. Serve with tahini dip.
4. Enjoy!

Nutritional Information (approximate): Calories per serving: 150; Protein: 4g; Fat: 12g; Saturated Fat: 2g; Carbohydrates: 10g; Fiber: 4g; Sugar: 4g; Sodium: 200mg

Tips and Variations:

- Add herbs like parsley or cilantro to the dip for extra flavor.
- Use other vegetables like bell peppers or cucumbers.
- Perfect for a healthy and refreshing snack.

Servings: 4

Cooking Time:

- **Prep Time:** 10 minutes
- **Cook Time:** 0 minutes
- **Total Time:** 10 minutes

Ingredients:

- 12 Medjool dates, pitted
- 12 almonds
- 2 tbsp almond butter

Instructions:

1. Make a small slit in each date and stuff with one almond.
2. Drizzle with almond butter.
3. Arrange on a plate and serve.
4. Enjoy!

Nutritional Information (approximate): Calories per serving: 180; Protein: 3g; Fat: 8g; Saturated Fat: 0.5g; Carbohydrates: 28g; Fiber: 4g; Sugar: 24g; Sodium: 5mg

Tips and Variations:

- Sprinkle with sea salt for a sweet and salty treat.
- Use other nuts like walnuts or pecans.
- Perfect for a quick and energy-boosting snack.

Servings: 4

Cooking Time:

- **Prep Time:** 10 minutes
- **Cook Time:** 20 minutes
- **Total Time:** 30 minutes

Ingredients:

- 1 bunch kale, stems removed and leaves torn into bite-sized pieces
- 2 tbsp olive oil
- 1/2 tsp sea salt

Instructions:

1. Preheat oven to 300°F (150°C).
2. In a large bowl, toss kale with olive oil and sea salt.
3. Spread kale in a single layer on a baking sheet.
4. Bake for 20 minutes, or until crispy, turning halfway through.
5. Allow to cool slightly before serving.
6. Enjoy!

Nutritional Information (approximate): Calories per serving: 100; Protein: 2g; Fat: 7g; Saturated Fat: 1g; Carbohydrates: 8g; Fiber: 2g; Sugar: 0g; Sodium: 150mg

Tips and Variations:

- Sprinkle with nutritional yeast for a cheesy flavor.
- Add spices like paprika or garlic powder.

Servings: 12 balls

Cooking Time:

- **Prep Time:** 15 minutes
- **Cook Time:** 0 minutes
- **Total Time:** 15 minutes

Ingredients:

- 1 cup dates, pitted
- 1/2 cup almonds
- 1/2 cup walnuts
- 1/4 cup dried cranberries
- 1/4 cup dried blueberries
- 2 tbsp chia seeds
- 1 tbsp honey
- 1 tsp vanilla extract

Instructions:

1. In a food processor, combine dates, almonds, and walnuts. Process until finely chopped.
2. Add dried cranberries, dried blueberries, chia seeds, honey, and vanilla extract. Process until mixture comes together.
3. Roll mixture into 1-inch balls.
4. Store in an airtight container in the refrigerator.
5. Enjoy!

Nutritional Information (approximate): Calories per ball: 90; Protein: 2g; Fat: 5g; Saturated Fat: 0.5g; Carbohydrates: 12g; Fiber: 2g; Sugar: 9g; Sodium: 0mg

Tips and Variations:

- Roll in shredded coconut for extra texture.
- Use other nuts or seeds according to preference.
- Perfect for a quick energy boost.

Avocado Deviled Eggs

Servings: 4

Cooking Time:

- **Prep Time:** 15 minutes
- **Cook Time:** 10 minutes
- **Total Time:** 25 minutes

Ingredients:

- 6 eggs
- 1 ripe avocado
- 1 tbsp lime juice
- 1 tbsp Greek yogurt
- 1/2 tsp garlic powder
- Salt and pepper, to taste
- Paprika, for garnish

Instructions:

1. Place eggs in a saucepan and cover with water. Bring to a boil, then reduce heat and simmer for 10 minutes.
2. Drain and transfer eggs to a bowl of ice water. Let cool for 5 minutes.
3. Peel eggs and slice in half lengthwise. Remove yolks and place in a bowl.
4. Add avocado, lime juice, Greek yogurt, garlic powder, salt, and pepper to the yolks. Mash until smooth.
5. Spoon or pipe the avocado mixture into the egg whites.

6. Sprinkle with paprika.
7. Serve immediately.
8. Enjoy!

Nutritional Information (approximate): Calories per serving: 120; Protein: 6g; Fat: 10g; Saturated Fat: 2g; Carbohydrates: 3g; Fiber: 2g; Sugar: 1g; Sodium: 150mg

Tips and Variations:

- Add chopped chives or green onions for extra flavor.
- Use lemon juice instead of lime for a different taste.
- Perfect for a healthy and protein-rich snack.

Servings: 12 bites

Cooking Time:

- **Prep Time:** 20 minutes
- **Cook Time:** 25 minutes
- **Total Time:** 45 minutes

Ingredients:

- 1 cup cooked quinoa
- 1/2 cup grated zucchini
- 1/2 cup grated carrot
- 1/4 cup chopped spinach
- 1/4 cup grated Parmesan cheese
- 1 egg
- 1/2 tsp garlic powder
- Salt and pepper, to taste
- Olive oil spray

Instructions:

1. Preheat oven to 375°F (190°C).
2. In a large bowl, combine cooked quinoa, grated zucchini, grated carrot, chopped spinach, Parmesan cheese, egg, garlic powder, salt, and pepper.
3. Mix until well combined.
4. Spray a mini muffin tin with olive oil spray. Spoon quinoa mixture into each cup, pressing down slightly.

5. Bake for 20-25 minutes, or until golden brown and set.

6. Allow to cool slightly before removing from the tin.

7. Serve warm or at room temperature.

8. Enjoy!

Nutritional Information (approximate): Calories per bite: 50; Protein: 2g; Fat: 2g; Saturated Fat: 0.5g; Carbohydrates: 6g; Fiber: 1g; Sugar: 1g; Sodium: 50mg

Tips and Variations:
- Add chopped herbs like parsley or cilantro for extra flavor.
- Use a different cheese like feta or cheddar.
- Perfect for a healthy and portable snack.

SAUCES, DRESSINGS, AND DIPS

Classic Hummus

Servings: 4

Cooking Time:

- **Prep Time:** 10 minutes
- **Cook Time:** 0 minutes
- **Total Time:** 10 minutes

Ingredients:

- 1 can chickpeas, drained and rinsed
- 1/4 cup tahini
- 2 tbsp olive oil
- 1 lemon, juiced
- 2 cloves garlic, minced
- 1/2 tsp ground cumin
- Salt, to taste
- 1/4 cup water (or as needed for consistency)

Instructions:

1. In a food processor, combine chickpeas, tahini, olive oil, lemon juice, garlic, cumin, and salt. Blend until smooth.
2. Add water, a tablespoon at a time, to reach desired consistency.
3. Serve with veggies, pita bread, or as a spread.
4. Enjoy!

Nutritional Information (approximate): Calories per serving: 200; Protein: 6g; Fat: 12g; Saturated Fat: 1.5g; Carbohydrates: 18g; Fiber: 6g; Sugar: 2g; Sodium: 300mg

Tips and Variations:

- Add roasted red peppers or sun-dried tomatoes to the hummus for extra flavor.
- Use as a spread for sandwiches or wraps.
- Store in the refrigerator for up to 5 days.

Avocado Cilantro Dressing

Servings: 4

Cooking Time:

- **Prep Time:** 10 minutes
- **Cook Time:** 0 minutes
- **Total Time:** 10 minutes

Ingredients:

- 1 ripe avocado
- 1/4 cup fresh cilantro
- 1/4 cup Greek yogurt
- 1 lime, juiced
- 1 clove garlic
- 2 tbsp olive oil

- Salt and pepper, to taste
- Water, as needed for consistency

Instructions:

1. In a blender, combine avocado, cilantro, Greek yogurt, lime juice, garlic, olive oil, salt, and pepper.
2. Blend until smooth, adding water as needed to reach desired consistency.
3. Serve over salads or as a dip for veggies.
4. Enjoy!

Nutritional Information (approximate): Calories per serving: 120; Protein: 2g; Fat: 11g; Saturated Fat: 2g; Carbohydrates: 6g; Fiber: 3g; Sugar: 1g; Sodium: 150mg

Tips and Variations:

- Add jalapeño for a spicy kick.
- Use as a spread for sandwiches or wraps.
- Store in an airtight container in the refrigerator for up to 3 days.

Servings: 4

Cooking Time:

- **Prep Time:** 5 minutes
- **Cook Time:** 0 minutes
- **Total Time:** 5 minutes

Ingredients:

- 1/4 cup tahini
- 1 lemon, juiced
- 1 clove garlic, minced
- 1/2 tsp ground turmeric
- 1/4 tsp ground cumin
- Salt and pepper, to taste
- Water, as needed for consistency

Instructions:

1. In a bowl, whisk together tahini, lemon juice, garlic, turmeric, cumin, salt, and pepper.
2. Add water, a tablespoon at a time, until desired consistency is reached.
3. Serve over roasted vegetables or as a dip.
4. Enjoy!

Nutritional Information (approximate): Calories per serving: 80; Protein: 3g; Fat: 6g; Saturated Fat: 1g; Carbohydrates: 5g; Fiber: 2g; Sugar: 0g; Sodium: 150mg

Tips and Variations:

- Add a pinch of cayenne pepper for extra heat.
- Use as a dressing for salads or grain bowls.
- Store in the refrigerator for up to 5 days.

Lemon Vinaigrette

Servings: 4

Cooking Time:

- **Prep Time:** 5 minutes
- **Cook Time:** 0 minutes
- **Total Time:** 5 minutes

Ingredients:

- 1/4 cup olive oil
- 1 lemon, juiced
- 1 tsp Dijon mustard
- 1 clove garlic, minced
- Salt and pepper, to taste

Instructions:

1. In a small bowl, whisk together olive oil, lemon juice, Dijon mustard, garlic, salt, and pepper.
2. Serve over salads or as a marinade for grilled vegetables.
3. Enjoy!

Nutritional Information (approximate): Calories per serving: 90; Protein: 0g; Fat: 9g; Saturated Fat: 1.5g; Carbohydrates: 2g; Fiber: 0g; Sugar: 0g; Sodium: 100mg

Tips and Variations:

- Add fresh herbs like parsley or basil for extra flavor.
- Use lime juice instead of lemon for a different taste.
- Store in the refrigerator for up to 1 week.

Servings: 4

Cooking Time:

- **Prep Time:** 10 minutes
- **Cook Time:** 0 minutes
- **Total Time:** 10 minutes

Ingredients:

- 2 cups fresh basil leaves
- 1/2 cup grated Parmesan cheese
- 1/3 cup pine nuts
- 2 cloves garlic
- 1/2 cup olive oil
- Salt and pepper, to taste

Instructions:

1. In a food processor, combine basil, Parmesan cheese, pine nuts, and garlic. Pulse until finely chopped.
2. With the processor running, slowly add olive oil until the mixture is smooth.
3. Season with salt and pepper to taste.
4. Serve over pasta, grilled vegetables, or as a spread.
5. Enjoy!

Nutritional Information (approximate): Calories per serving: 200; Protein: 4g; Fat: 20g; Saturated Fat: 3g; Carbohydrates: 2g; Fiber: 1g; Sugar: 0g; Sodium: 150mg

Tips and Variations:

- Use walnuts or almonds instead of pine nuts.
- Add spinach or arugula for a different flavor.
- Store in the refrigerator for up to 5 days.

Cucumber Dill Dip

Servings: 4

Cooking Time:

- **Prep Time:** 10 minutes
- **Cook Time:** 0 minutes
- **Total Time:** 10 minutes

Ingredients:

- 1 cup Greek yogurt
- 1/2 cucumber, finely chopped
- 2 tbsp fresh dill, chopped
- 1 clove garlic, minced
- 1 tbsp lemon juice
- Salt and pepper, to taste

Instructions:

1. In a bowl, combine Greek yogurt, cucumber, dill, garlic, lemon juice, salt, and pepper. Mix well.
2. Serve with veggies, pita bread, or as a spread.
3. Enjoy!

Nutritional Information (approximate): Calories per serving: 50; Protein: 5g; Fat: 2g; Saturated Fat: 1g; Carbohydrates: 3g; Fiber: 0g; Sugar: 2g; Sodium: 50mg

Tips and Variations:

- Add fresh mint for extra flavor.
- Use as a sauce for grilled meats or fish.
- Store in the refrigerator for up to 3 days.

Servings: 4

Cooking Time:

- **Prep Time:** 5 minutes
- **Cook Time:** 0 minutes
- **Total Time:** 5 minutes

Ingredients:

- 1/4 cup peanut butter
- 2 tbsp soy sauce or tamari
- 1 tbsp rice vinegar
- 1 tbsp honey
- 1 clove garlic, minced
- 1 tsp grated ginger
- 1-2 tbsp water (as needed for consistency)
- 1/4 tsp red pepper flakes (optional)

Instructions:

1. In a bowl, whisk together peanut butter, soy sauce, rice vinegar, honey, garlic, ginger, and red pepper flakes (if using).
2. Add water, a tablespoon at a time, until desired consistency is reached.
3. Serve as a dip, dressing, or sauce.
4. Enjoy!

Nutritional Information (approximate): Calories per serving: 120; Protein: 4g; Fat: 8g; Saturated Fat: 2g; Carbohydrates: 8g; Fiber: 1g; Sugar: 5g; Sodium: 300mg

Tips and Variations:

- Use almond butter instead of peanut butter.
- Add a splash of lime juice for extra tang.
- Store in the refrigerator for up to 5 days.

Mango Salsa

Servings: 4

Cooking Time:

- **Prep Time:** 10 minutes
- **Cook Time:** 0 minutes
- **Total Time:** 10 minutes

Ingredients:

- 2 ripe mangoes, diced
- 1 red bell pepper, diced
- 1/2 red onion, finely chopped
- 1 jalapeño, minced (optional)
- 1/4 cup fresh cilantro, chopped
- 1 lime, juiced
- Salt and pepper, to taste

Instructions:

1. In a bowl, combine mangoes, red bell pepper, red onion, jalapeño, cilantro, lime juice, salt, and pepper. Mix well.
2. Serve with tortilla chips, grilled meats, or fish.
3. Enjoy!

Nutritional Information (approximate): Calories per serving: 60; Protein: 1g; Fat: 0.5g; Saturated Fat: 0g; Carbohydrates: 15g; Fiber: 2g; Sugar: 13g; Sodium: 5mg

Tips and Variations:

- Add diced avocado for extra creaminess.
- Use pineapple instead of mango for a different flavor.
- Store in the refrigerator for up to 2 days.

Servings: 4

Cooking Time:

- **Prep Time:** 5 minutes
- **Cook Time:** 0 minutes
- **Total Time:** 5 minutes

Ingredients:

- 1/2 cup mayonnaise
- 1 clove garlic, minced
- 1 tbsp lemon juice
- 1 tbsp fresh parsley, chopped
- 1 tsp Dijon mustard
- Salt and pepper, to taste

Instructions:

1. In a bowl, combine mayonnaise, garlic, lemon juice, parsley, Dijon mustard, salt, and pepper. Mix well.
2. Serve as a dip, spread, or sauce.
3. Enjoy!

Nutritional Information (approximate): Calories per serving: 150; Protein: 0g; Fat: 16g; Saturated Fat: 3g; Carbohydrates: 1g; Fiber: 0g; Sugar: 0g; Sodium: 200mg

Tips and Variations:

- Add other herbs like basil or dill for extra flavor.
- Use Greek yogurt instead of mayonnaise for a lighter version.
- Store in the refrigerator for up to 1 week.

Cashew Cream

Servings: 4

Cooking Time:

- **Prep Time:** 10 minutes (plus soaking time)
- **Cook Time:** 0 minutes
- **Total Time:** 10 minutes

Ingredients:

- 1 cup raw cashews, soaked overnight
- 1/2 cup water
- 1 tbsp lemon juice
- 1 clove garlic (optional)
- Salt, to taste

Instructions:

1. Drain and rinse the soaked cashews.
2. In a blender, combine cashews, water, lemon juice, garlic (if using), and salt. Blend until smooth.
3. Serve as a dip, sauce, or spread.
4. Enjoy!

Nutritional Information (approximate): Calories per serving: 120; Protein: 3g; Fat: 10g; Saturated Fat: 2g; Carbohydrates: 6g; Fiber: 1g; Sugar: 1g; Sodium: 5mg

Tips and Variations:

- Add nutritional yeast for a cheesy flavor.
- Use as a base for creamy dressings or sauces.
- Store in the refrigerator for up to 5 days.

Chimichurri Sauce

Servings: 4

Cooking Time:

- **Prep Time:** 10 minutes
- **Cook Time:** 0 minutes
- **Total Time:** 10 minutes

Ingredients:

- 1 cup fresh parsley, chopped
- 1/4 cup fresh cilantro, chopped
- 1/2 cup olive oil
- 1/4 cup red wine vinegar
- 2 cloves garlic, minced

- 1 tsp red pepper flakes (optional)
- Salt and pepper, to taste

Instructions:

1. In a bowl, combine parsley, cilantro, olive oil, red wine vinegar, garlic, red pepper flakes, salt, and pepper. Mix well.
2. Serve over grilled meats or vegetables.
3. Enjoy!

Nutritional Information (approximate): Calories per serving: 200; Protein: 1g; Fat: 21g; Saturated Fat: 3g; Carbohydrates: 2g; Fiber: 1g; Sugar: 0g; Sodium: 50mg

Tips and Variations:

- Add oregano for extra flavor.
- Use as a marinade for meats or vegetables.
- Store in the refrigerator for up to 1 week.

Servings: 4

Cooking Time:

- **Prep Time:** 5 minutes
- **Cook Time:** 0 minutes
- **Total Time:** 5 minutes

Ingredients:

- 1/4 cup Dijon mustard
- 2 tbsp honey
- 2 tbsp apple cider vinegar
- 1/4 cup olive oil
- Salt and pepper, to taste

Instructions:

1. In a small bowl, whisk together Dijon mustard, honey, apple cider vinegar, olive oil, salt, and pepper.
2. Serve over salads or as a dip for chicken tenders.
3. Enjoy!

Nutritional Information (approximate): Calories per serving: 130; Protein: 0g; Fat: 11g; Saturated Fat: 1.5g; Carbohydrates: 9g; Fiber: 0g; Sugar: 8g; Sodium: 200mg

Tips and Variations:

- Add a pinch of cayenne pepper for extra heat.
- Use whole grain mustard for a different texture.
- Store in the refrigerator for up to 1 week.

Servings: 4

Cooking Time:

- **Prep Time:** 5 minutes
- **Cook Time:** 0 minutes
- **Total Time:** 5 minutes

Ingredients:

- 2 tbsp white miso paste
- 2 tbsp rice vinegar
- 1 tbsp soy sauce or tamari
- 1 tbsp sesame oil
- 1 tbsp grated ginger
- 1 tsp honey
- Water, as needed for consistency

Instructions:

1. In a bowl, whisk together miso paste, rice vinegar, soy sauce, sesame oil, grated ginger, honey, and water until smooth.
2. Serve over salads or as a dip for vegetables.
3. Enjoy!

Nutritional Information (approximate): Calories per serving: 80; Protein: 2g; Fat: 5g; Saturated Fat: 1g; Carbohydrates: 6g; Fiber: 0g; Sugar: 4g; Sodium: 400mg

Tips and Variations:

- Add garlic for extra flavor.
- Use as a marinade for tofu or chicken.
- Store in the refrigerator for up to 1 week.

Coconut Curry Sauce

Servings: 4

Cooking Time:

- **Prep Time:** 5 minutes
- **Cook Time:** 15 minutes
- **Total Time:** 20 minutes

Ingredients:

- 1 can coconut milk
- 2 tbsp red curry paste
- 1 tbsp fish sauce (or soy sauce for vegetarian)
- 1 tbsp lime juice
- 1 tbsp brown sugar
- 1 clove garlic, minced
- 1 tsp grated ginger

Instructions:

1. In a saucepan, combine coconut milk, red curry paste, fish sauce, lime juice, brown sugar, garlic, and ginger.

2. Bring to a simmer over medium heat, stirring frequently.

3. Simmer for 10-15 minutes, until the sauce thickens slightly.

4. Serve over rice, noodles, or as a sauce for vegetables or protein.

5. Enjoy!

Nutritional Information (approximate): Calories per serving: 250; Protein: 3g; Fat: 22g; Saturated Fat: 19g; Carbohydrates: 10g; Fiber: 1g; Sugar: 6g; Sodium: 600mg

Tips and Variations:
- Add fresh basil or cilantro for extra flavor.
- Use as a base for soups or stews.
- Store in the refrigerator for up to 1 week.

DESSERTS AND SWEET TREATS

Dark Chocolate Avocado Mousse

Servings: 4

Cooking Time:

- **Prep Time:** 10 minutes
- **Cook Time:** 0 minutes
- **Total Time:** 10 minutes

Ingredients:

- 2 ripe avocados
- 1/2 cup cocoa powder
- 1/4 cup maple syrup
- 1/4 cup almond milk (or other plant-based milk)
- 1 tsp vanilla extract
- Pinch of salt
- Fresh berries (optional, for garnish)

Instructions:

1. In a blender or food processor, combine avocados, cocoa powder, maple syrup, almond milk, vanilla extract, and salt. Blend until smooth and creamy.
2. Taste and adjust sweetness if necessary.
3. Divide into serving bowls and refrigerate for at least 30 minutes before serving.

4. Garnish with fresh berries if desired.

5. Enjoy!

Nutritional Information (approximate): Calories per serving: 200; Protein: 3g; Fat: 15g; Saturated Fat: 2.5g; Carbohydrates: 18g; Fiber: 7g; Sugar: 10g; Sodium: 60mg

Tips and Variations:

- Add a pinch of cinnamon or chili powder for extra flavor.
- Top with coconut whipped cream for added indulgence.
- Store in the refrigerator for up to 2 days.

Coconut Macaroons

Servings: 12

Cooking Time:

- **Prep Time:** 10 minutes
- **Cook Time:** 20 minutes
- **Total Time:** 30 minutes

Ingredients:

- 2 cups shredded coconut (unsweetened)
- 1/4 cup coconut flour
- 1/4 cup maple syrup
- 2 tbsp coconut oil, melted

- 1 tsp vanilla extract
- Pinch of salt

Instructions:

1. Preheat oven to 325°F (160°C). Line a baking sheet with parchment paper.
2. In a bowl, combine shredded coconut, coconut flour, maple syrup, melted coconut oil, vanilla extract, and salt. Mix well.
3. Using a small cookie scoop or spoon, form mixture into balls and place on the prepared baking sheet.
4. Bake for 15-20 minutes, or until golden brown.
5. Let cool on the baking sheet before transferring to a wire rack.
6. Enjoy!

Nutritional Information (approximate): Calories per serving: 90; Protein: 1g; Fat: 8g; Saturated Fat: 7g; Carbohydrates: 6g; Fiber: 2g; Sugar: 4g; Sodium: 15mg

Tips and Variations:

- Dip the bottoms in melted dark chocolate for a decadent treat.
- Add a touch of almond extract for a different flavor.
- Store in an airtight container for up to 1 week.

Servings: 4

Cooking Time:

- **Prep Time:** 5 minutes (plus freezing time)
- **Cook Time:** 0 minutes
- **Total Time:** 5 minutes

Ingredients:

- 4 ripe bananas, sliced and frozen
- 1 tsp vanilla extract
- Optional mix-ins: cocoa powder, peanut butter, berries, nuts

Instructions:

1. In a blender or food processor, blend frozen banana slices until smooth and creamy.
2. Add vanilla extract and blend again.
3. Serve immediately or freeze for a firmer texture.
4. Enjoy!

Nutritional Information (approximate): Calories per serving: 90; Protein: 1g; Fat: 0g; Saturated Fat: 0g; Carbohydrates: 23g; Fiber: 3g; Sugar: 12g; Sodium: 0mg

Tips and Variations:

- Add cocoa powder for chocolate banana ice cream.
- Mix in peanut butter for a creamy twist.

Servings: 12

Cooking Time:

- **Prep Time:** 10 minutes
- **Cook Time:** 25 minutes
- **Total Time:** 35 minutes

Ingredients:

- 1 cup almond flour
- 1/2 cup cocoa powder
- 1/2 cup coconut sugar
- 1/4 cup coconut oil, melted
- 3 eggs
- 1 tsp vanilla extract
- 1/2 tsp baking soda
- Pinch of salt
- 1/2 cup dark chocolate chips (optional)

Instructions:

1. Preheat oven to 350°F (175°C). Line an 8x8-inch baking pan with parchment paper.
2. In a bowl, combine almond flour, cocoa powder, coconut sugar, and salt. Mix well.
3. In a separate bowl, whisk together melted coconut oil, eggs, and vanilla extract.

4. Add the wet ingredients to the dry ingredients and mix until combined. Fold in dark chocolate chips if using.

5. Pour the batter into the prepared baking pan and spread evenly.

6. Bake for 20-25 minutes, or until a toothpick inserted into the center comes out clean.

7. Let cool completely before cutting into squares.

8. Enjoy!

Nutritional Information (approximate): Calories per serving: 150; Protein: 4g; Fat: 12g; Saturated Fat: 5g; Carbohydrates: 11g; Fiber: 2g; Sugar: 7g; Sodium: 70mg

Tips and Variations:
- Add chopped nuts for extra crunch.
- Substitute maple syrup for coconut sugar if preferred.
- Store in an airtight container for up to 5 days.

Servings: 6

Cooking Time:

- **Prep Time:** 15 minutes
- **Cook Time:** 30 minutes
- **Total Time:** 45 minutes

Ingredients:

- 4 cups mixed berries (blueberries, raspberries, strawberries)
- 2 tbsp maple syrup
- 1 tbsp lemon juice
- 1 tsp vanilla extract
- 1 cup almond flour
- 1/2 cup rolled oats (gluten-free if necessary)
- 1/4 cup coconut sugar
- 1/4 cup coconut oil, melted
- 1/2 tsp cinnamon
- Pinch of salt

Instructions:

1. Preheat oven to 350°F (175°C). Grease a baking dish.
2. In a bowl, combine mixed berries, maple syrup, lemon juice, and vanilla extract. Transfer to the prepared baking dish.
3. In another bowl, mix almond flour, rolled oats, coconut sugar, melted coconut oil, cinnamon, and salt until crumbly.

4. Sprinkle the crumble mixture evenly over the berries.

5. Bake for 25-30 minutes, or until the topping is golden brown and the berries are bubbling.

6. Let cool slightly before serving.

7. Enjoy!

Nutritional Information (approximate): Calories per serving: 200; Protein: 3g; Fat: 12g; Saturated Fat: 6g; Carbohydrates: 23g; Fiber: 5g; Sugar: 14g; Sodium: 20mg

Tips and Variations:

- Serve with a dollop of coconut yogurt or whipped cream.
- Add chopped nuts to the crumble for extra texture.
- Store leftovers in the refrigerator for up to 3 days.

Servings: 12

Cooking Time:

- **Prep Time:** 10 minutes
- **Cook Time:** 0 minutes
- **Total Time:** 10 minutes

Ingredients:

- 1 cup rolled oats (gluten-free if necessary)
- 1/2 cup pumpkin puree
- 1/4 cup almond butter
- 1/4 cup maple syrup
- 1/4 cup ground flaxseed
- 1 tsp pumpkin pie spice
- 1/2 tsp vanilla extract
- Pinch of salt

Instructions:

1. In a bowl, combine rolled oats, pumpkin puree, almond butter, maple syrup, ground flaxseed, pumpkin pie spice, vanilla extract, and salt. Mix until well combined.
2. Using a tablespoon, scoop the mixture and roll into balls.
3. Place the energy balls on a baking sheet and refrigerate for at least 30 minutes to firm up.
4. Store in an airtight container in the refrigerator.

5. Enjoy!

Nutritional Information (approximate): Calories per serving: 90; Protein: 2g; Fat: 4g; Saturated Fat: 0.5g; Carbohydrates: 12g; Fiber: 2g; Sugar: 5g; Sodium: 10mg

Tips and Variations:
- Add mini chocolate chips for a sweet twist.
- Roll the balls in shredded coconut or crushed nuts for extra flavor.
- Store in the refrigerator for up to 1 week.

Servings: 4

Cooking Time:

- **Prep Time:** 10 minutes
- **Cook Time:** 30 minutes
- **Total Time:** 40 minutes

Ingredients:

- 4 large apples, cored
- 1/4 cup chopped nuts (walnuts, pecans)
- 2 tbsp raisins
- 2 tbsp maple syrup
- 1 tsp cinnamon
- 1/4 tsp nutmeg
- 1/4 cup water

Instructions:

1. Preheat oven to 375°F (190°C). Grease a baking dish. 2. In a small bowl, combine chopped nuts, raisins, maple syrup, cinnamon, and nutmeg.
3. Stuff each cored apple with the nut mixture, packing it tightly.
4. Place the stuffed apples in the prepared baking dish.
5. Pour water into the bottom of the dish.
6. Cover the dish with foil and bake for 20-25 minutes.

7. Remove the foil and bake for an additional 5-10 minutes, or until the apples are tender.

8. Serve warm, optionally with a scoop of vanilla yogurt or a drizzle of honey.

9. Enjoy!

Nutritional Information (approximate): Calories per serving: 150; Protein: 2g; Fat: 5g; Saturated Fat: 0.5g; Carbohydrates: 30g; Fiber: 5g; Sugar: 20g; Sodium: 0mg

Tips and Variations:

- Experiment with different types of apples for varied flavors and textures.
- Add a sprinkle of granola on top before serving for extra crunch.
- Serve with a scoop of vanilla ice cream for a decadent dessert.

Servings: 12

Cooking Time:

- **Prep Time:** 10 minutes
- **Cook Time:** 0 minutes
- **Total Time:** 10 minutes

Ingredients:

- 1 cup rolled oats
- 1/4 cup almond butter
- 2 tbsp maple syrup
- 1 tbsp matcha powder
- 1/4 cup shredded coconut (unsweetened)
- 1/4 cup chopped nuts (such as almonds or cashews)
- 1/4 cup dried cranberries (or other dried fruit)
- 1 tsp vanilla extract
- Pinch of salt

Instructions:

1. In a bowl, combine rolled oats, almond butter, maple syrup, matcha powder, shredded coconut, chopped nuts, dried cranberries, vanilla extract, and salt. Mix until well combined.
2. Using a tablespoon, scoop the mixture and roll into balls.
3. Place the energy bites on a baking sheet and refrigerate for at least 30 minutes to firm up.

4. Store in an airtight container in the refrigerator.

5. Enjoy!

Nutritional Information (approximate): Calories per serving: 90; Protein: 2g; Fat: 4g; Saturated Fat: 1g; Carbohydrates: 12g; Fiber: 2g; Sugar: 5g; Sodium: 10mg

Tips and Variations:

- Add a tablespoon of chia seeds for extra fiber and omega-3 fatty acids.
- Roll the energy bites in matcha powder for an extra boost of green tea flavor.
- Store in the refrigerator for up to 1 week.

Servings: 12

Cooking Time:

- **Prep Time:** 10 minutes
- **Cook Time:** 10 minutes
- **Total Time:** 20 minutes

Ingredients:

- 1 cup dark chocolate chips
- 1/4 cup peanut butter
- 1/4 cup chopped nuts (such as almonds or peanuts)
- 1/4 cup dried fruit (such as cranberries or raisins)
- Pinch of sea salt

Instructions:

1. Line a baking sheet with parchment paper.
2. In a microwave-safe bowl, melt the dark chocolate chips in 30-second intervals, stirring in between, until smooth.
3. Spread the melted chocolate evenly onto the prepared baking sheet.
4. In a separate microwave-safe bowl, melt the peanut butter until smooth.
5. Drizzle the melted peanut butter over the chocolate layer.
6. Using a toothpick or knife, swirl the peanut butter into the chocolate to create a marbled effect.
7. Sprinkle chopped nuts, dried fruit, and sea salt over the top.

8. Place the baking sheet in the refrigerator for 1-2 hours, or until the bark is firm.

9. Once set, break the bark into pieces.

10.   Store in an airtight container in the refrigerator.

11. Enjoy!

Nutritional Information (approximate): Calories per serving: 150; Protein: 3g; Fat: 10g; Saturated Fat: 4g; Carbohydrates: 13g; Fiber: 2g; Sugar: 9g; Sodium: 50mg

Tips and Variations:

- Use almond butter or cashew butter instead of peanut butter for a different flavor.
- Experiment with different toppings like shredded coconut or crushed pretzels.
- Store in the refrigerator for up to 2 weeks.

Servings: 12

Cooking Time:

- **Prep Time:** 10 minutes
- **Cook Time:** 0 minutes
- **Total Time:** 10 minutes

Ingredients:

- 1 cup shredded coconut (unsweetened), plus extra for rolling
- 1/4 cup almond flour
- Zest of 1 lemon
- 2 tbsp lemon juice
- 2 tbsp maple syrup
- 1/2 tsp vanilla extract
- Pinch of salt

Instructions:

1. In a food processor, combine shredded coconut, almond flour, lemon zest, lemon juice, maple syrup, vanilla extract, and salt. Pulse until the mixture comes together and forms a dough.
2. Using a tablespoon, scoop the mixture and roll into balls.
3. Roll the balls in additional shredded coconut to coat.
4. Place the bliss balls on a baking sheet and refrigerate for at least 30 minutes to firm up.

5. Store in an airtight container in the refrigerator.

6. Enjoy!

Nutritional Information (approximate): Calories per serving: 90; Protein: 1g; Fat: 7g; Saturated Fat: 6g; Carbohydrates: 7g; Fiber: 2g; Sugar: 4g; Sodium: 10mg

Tips and Variations:

- Add a teaspoon of chia seeds for extra fiber and omega-3 fatty acids.
- Substitute lime juice for lemon juice for a different citrus flavor.
- Store in the refrigerator for up to 1 week.

Servings: 12

Cooking Time:

- **Prep Time:** 20 minutes
- **Cook Time:** 30 minutes
- **Total Time:** 50 minutes

Ingredients:

For the Raspberry Chia Jam:

- 2 cups fresh or frozen raspberries
- 2 tbsp maple syrup
- 2 tbsp chia seeds
- 1 tsp lemon juice

For the Oat Crust:

- 1 1/2 cups rolled oats
- 1/2 cup almond flour
- 1/4 cup coconut oil, melted
- 1/4 cup maple syrup
- 1 tsp vanilla extract
- Pinch of salt

Instructions:

1. Preheat oven to 350°F (175°C). Grease an 8x8-inch baking pan.

2. In a saucepan, combine raspberries and maple syrup. Cook over medium heat, stirring occasionally, until raspberries break down and become syrupy, about 5-7 minutes.

3. Remove from heat and stir in chia seeds and lemon juice. Let cool and thicken for about 10 minutes.

4. In a mixing bowl, combine rolled oats, almond flour, melted coconut oil, maple syrup, vanilla extract, and salt. Mix until well combined and crumbly.

5. Press half of the oat mixture firmly into the bottom of the prepared baking pan to form the crust.

6. Spread the raspberry chia jam evenly over the oat crust.

7. Sprinkle the remaining oat mixture over the top of the jam layer, pressing lightly to adhere.

8. Bake for 25-30 minutes, or until the top is golden brown.

9. Let cool completely before cutting into bars.Enjoy!

Nutritional Information (approximate): Calories per serving: 150; Protein: 3g; Fat: 7g; Saturated Fat: 3g; Carbohydrates: 20g; Fiber: 4g; Sugar: 8g; Sodium: 20mg

Tips and Variations:

- Substitute other berries like strawberries or blackberries for a different flavor.
- Add a sprinkle of shredded coconut or chopped nuts to the oat mixture for extra texture.
- Store leftovers in an airtight container in the refrigerator for up to 1 week.

Servings: 4

Cooking Time:

- **Prep Time:** 5 minutes (plus freezing time)
- **Cook Time:** 0 minutes
- **Total Time:** 5 minutes

Ingredients:

- 2 ripe mangos, peeled and chopped
- 1/4 cup coconut milk (or other plant-based milk)
- 2 tbsp maple syrup (optional)
- Juice of 1 lime
- Pinch of salt

Instructions:

1. Place chopped mangos in a blender or food processor.
2. Add coconut milk, maple syrup (if using), lime juice, and salt.
3. Blend until smooth and creamy.
4. Taste and adjust sweetness, if necessary, by adding more maple syrup.
5. Pour the mixture into a shallow dish and freeze for at least 4 hours, or until firm.
6. Once frozen, let the sorbet sit at room temperature for a few minutes to soften slightly.

7. Scoop into bowls and serve immediately.

8. Enjoy!

Nutritional Information (approximate): Calories per serving: 100; Protein: 1g; Fat: 2g; Saturated Fat: 2g; Carbohydrates: 23g; Fiber: 3g; Sugar: 19g; Sodium: 5mg

Tips and Variations:

- Add a splash of rum or vodka for an adult version.
- Mix in other fruits like pineapple or passionfruit for a tropical twist.
- Store leftover sorbet in an airtight container in the freezer for up to 2 weeks.

Servings: 2

Cooking Time:

- **Prep Time:** 5 minutes
- **Cook Time:** 0 minutes
- **Total Time:** 5 minutes

Ingredients:

- 1 cup coconut yogurt (unsweetened)
- 1 cup fresh fruit (such as berries, sliced bananas, or chopped mango)
- 2 tbsp shredded coconut (unsweetened)
- Drizzle of honey (optional)

Instructions:

1. Divide coconut yogurt between serving bowls.
2. Top with fresh fruit and shredded coconut.
3. Drizzle with honey if desired.
4. Serve immediately.
5. Enjoy!

Nutritional Information (approximate): Calories per serving: 150; Protein: 2g; Fat: 7g; Saturated Fat: 6g; Carbohydrates: 20g; Fiber: 4g; Sugar: 14g; Sodium: 20mg

Tips and Variations:

- Use dairy-based yogurt if preferred.
- Add a sprinkle of granola or nuts for extra crunch.
- Customize with your favorite fruits and toppings.

Blueberry Oat Muffins

Servings: 12 muffins

Cooking Time:

- **Prep Time:** 10 minutes
- **Cook Time:** 20 minutes
- **Total Time:** 30 minutes

Ingredients:

- 1 1/2 cups rolled oats
- 1 cup almond flour
- 1 tsp baking powder
- 1/2 tsp baking soda
- 1/2 tsp cinnamon
- Pinch of salt
- 2 ripe bananas, mashed
- 2 eggs
- 1/4 cup maple syrup
- 1/4 cup almond milk (or other plant-based milk)
- 1 tsp vanilla extract
- 1 cup fresh or frozen blueberries

Instructions:

1. Preheat oven to 350°F (175°C). Grease a muffin tin or line with paper liners.
2. In a blender or food processor, pulse rolled oats until finely ground to make oat flour.
3. In a large bowl, combine oat flour, almond flour, baking powder, baking soda, cinnamon, and salt.
4. In another bowl, whisk together mashed bananas, eggs, maple syrup, almond milk, and vanilla extract.
5. Pour the wet ingredients into the dry ingredients and stir until just combined.
6. Gently fold in blueberries.
7. Divide the batter evenly among the muffin cups.
8. Bake for 18-20 minutes, or until a toothpick inserted into the center comes out clean.
9. Let cool in the muffin tin for 5 minutes before transferring to a wire rack to cool completely. Enjoy!

Nutritional Information (approximate): Calories per serving: 150; Protein: 4g; Fat: 6g; Saturated Fat: 1g; Carbohydrates: 21g; Fiber: 3g; Sugar: 9g; Sodium: 100mg

Tips and Variations:

- Add a handful of chopped nuts or seeds for extra texture.
- Substitute other berries like raspberries or strawberries if desired.
- Store leftovers in an airtight container at room temperature for up to 3 days, or freeze for longer storage.

BEVERAGES AND SMOOTHIES

Green Detox Smoothie

Servings: 2

Prep Time: 5 minutes

Cook Time: 0 minutes

Total Time: 5 minutes

Ingredients:

- 2 cups spinach leaves
- 1 cucumber, peeled and chopped
- 1 green apple, cored and chopped
- 1/2 lemon, juiced
- 1-inch piece of ginger, peeled
- 1 cup coconut water
- Handful of ice cubes

Instructions:

1. Place all ingredients in a blender.
2. Blend until smooth and creamy.
3. Taste and adjust sweetness if needed.
4. Serve immediately.
5. Enjoy!

Nutritional Information (approximate): Calories per serving: 80; Protein: 2g; Fat: 0.5g; Saturated Fat: 0g; Carbohydrates: 20g; Fiber: 5g; Sugar: 12g; Sodium: 200mg

Tips and Variations:

- Add a handful of fresh mint leaves for extra freshness.
- Substitute kale or Swiss chard for spinach.
- Add a tablespoon of chia seeds for added protein and fiber.

Turmeric Golden Milk

Servings: 2
Prep Time: 5 minutes
Cook Time: 5 minutes
Total Time: 10 minutes

Ingredients:

- 2 cups unsweetened almond milk (or other plant-based milk)
- 1 tsp ground turmeric
- 1/2 tsp ground cinnamon
- 1/4 tsp ground ginger
- Pinch of black pepper
- 1 tbsp maple syrup or honey (optional)
- 1/2 tsp vanilla extract

Instructions:

1. In a small saucepan, heat almond milk over medium heat until warmed but not boiling.

2. Whisk in ground turmeric, cinnamon, ginger, black pepper, maple syrup or honey (if using), and vanilla extract.

3. Continue to cook for 3-5 minutes, stirring occasionally, until flavors are well combined.

4. Remove from heat and pour into mugs.

5. Serve warm.

6. Enjoy!

Nutritional Information (approximate): Calories per serving: 50; Protein: 1g; Fat: 2g; Saturated Fat: 0g; Carbohydrates: 7g; Fiber: 1g; Sugar: 5g; Sodium: 180mg

Tips and Variations:

- Add a pinch of ground nutmeg or cardamom for extra flavor.
- Use fresh turmeric root instead of ground turmeric for a more intense flavor.
- Adjust sweetness to taste with additional maple syrup or honey.

Servings: 2

Prep Time: 5 minutes

Cook Time: 0 minutes

Total Time: 5 minutes

Ingredients:

- 1 ripe banana
- 1 cup mixed berries (such as strawberries, blueberries, raspberries)
- 1/2 cup Greek yogurt
- 1/2 cup almond milk (or other plant-based milk)
- Handful of ice cubes
- Optional: 1 tbsp honey or maple syrup

Instructions:

1. Place all ingredients in a blender.
2. Blend until smooth and creamy.
3. Taste and adjust sweetness if needed.
4. Serve immediately.
5. Enjoy!

Nutritional Information (approximate): Calories per serving: 120; Protein: 5g; Fat: 2g; Saturated Fat: 0.5g; Carbohydrates: 22g; Fiber: 4g; Sugar: 14g; Sodium: 50mg

Tips and Variations:

- Use frozen berries for a thicker, colder smoothie.
- Add a handful of spinach or kale for extra nutrients.
- Substitute dairy-free yogurt for Greek yogurt for a vegan option.

Coconut Water with Lime and Mint

Servings: 2

Prep Time: 5 minutes

Cook Time: 0 minutes

Total Time: 5 minutes

Ingredients:

- 2 cups coconut water
- Juice of 1 lime
- Handful of fresh mint leaves
- Ice cubes (optional)

Instructions:

1. In a pitcher, combine coconut water and lime juice.
2. Add fresh mint leaves and stir gently.
3. Let it sit for a few minutes to allow the flavors to infuse.
4. Serve over ice if desired.
5. Enjoy!

Nutritional Information (approximate): Calories per serving: 25; Protein: 0g; Fat: 0g; Saturated Fat: 0g; Carbohydrates: 6g; Fiber: 0g; Sugar: 4g; Sodium: 60mg

Tips and Variations:

- Add slices of fresh cucumber for extra freshness.
- Use sparkling coconut water for a fizzy twist.
- Garnish with lime wedges and additional mint leaves for a decorative touch.

Matcha Latte

Servings: 1
Prep Time: 5 minutes
Cook Time: 5 minutes
Total Time: 10 minutes

Ingredients:

- 1 tsp matcha powder
- 1 cup unsweetened almond milk (or other plant-based milk)
- 1 tsp honey or maple syrup (optional)
- 1/2 tsp vanilla extract

Instructions:

1. In a small saucepan, heat almond milk over medium heat until warmed but not boiling.

2. In a mug, whisk matcha powder with a small amount of hot water until smooth and lump-free.

3. Pour the matcha mixture into the warmed almond milk.

4. Add honey or maple syrup (if using) and vanilla extract.

5. Whisk until well combined and frothy.

6. Pour into a mug and serve hot.

7. Enjoy!

Nutritional Information (approximate): Calories per serving: 30; Protein: 1g; Fat: 1g; Saturated Fat: 0g; Carbohydrates: 5g; Fiber: 1g; Sugar: 3g; Sodium: 150mg

Tips and Variations:
- Adjust sweetness to taste by adding more or less honey or maple syrup.
- Use a milk frother to create extra frothiness.
- Garnish with a sprinkle of matcha powder or cinnamon for a decorative touch.

Servings: 2

Prep Time: 5 minutes

Cook Time: 5 minutes

Total Time: 10 minutes

Ingredients:

- 2 cups water
- 1-inch piece of ginger, sliced
- 1 lemon, sliced
- 1-2 tbsp honey (optional)

Instructions:

1. In a small saucepan, bring water to a boil.
2. Add sliced ginger and lemon to the boiling water.
3. Reduce heat and simmer for 5 minutes.
4. Remove from heat and let it steep for a few more minutes.
5. Strain the tea into mugs.
6. Stir in honey if desired.
7. Serve hot.
8. Enjoy!

Nutritional Information (approximate): Calories per serving: 20; Protein: 0g; Fat: 0g; Saturated Fat: 0g; Carbohydrates: 6g; Fiber: 1g; Sugar: 4g; Sodium: 10mg

Tips and Variations:

- Add a cinnamon stick or a few cloves for extra flavor.
- Serve with a slice of fresh lemon or a sprig of mint for garnish.
- Enjoy cold as a refreshing iced tea on hot days.

Pumpkin Spice Smoothie

Servings: 2

Prep Time: 5 minutes

Cook Time: 0 minutes

Total Time: 5 minutes

Ingredients:

- 1 cup pumpkin puree
- 1 ripe banana
- 1 cup unsweetened almond milk (or other plant-based milk)
- 1/2 tsp pumpkin pie spice
- 1 tbsp maple syrup (optional)
- Handful of ice cubes

Instructions:

1. Place all ingredients in a blender.
2. Blend until smooth and creamy.
3. Taste and adjust sweetness if needed.
4. Serve immediately.

5. Enjoy!

Nutritional Information (approximate): Calories per serving: 100; Protein: 2g; Fat: 2g; Saturated Fat: 0g; Carbohydrates: 22g; Fiber: 4g; Sugar: 10g; Sodium: 80mg

Tips and Variations:
- Add a scoop of protein powder for an extra protein boost.
- Top with a dollop of whipped cream and a sprinkle of cinnamon for a decadent treat.
- Use frozen banana for a thicker, creamier smoothie.

Mango Pineapple Smoothie

Servings: 2
Prep Time: 5 minutes
Cook Time: 0 minutes
Total Time: 5 minutes

Ingredients:
- 1 cup chopped mango (fresh or frozen)
- 1 cup chopped pineapple (fresh or frozen)
- 1/2 cup Greek yogurt
- 1/2 cup coconut water or pineapple juice
- Handful of ice cubes (if using fresh fruit)

Instructions:

1. Place all ingredients in a blender.
2. Blend until smooth and creamy.
3. Taste and adjust sweetness if needed.
4. Serve immediately.
5. Enjoy!

Nutritional Information (approximate): Calories per serving: 120; Protein: 4g; Fat: 0.5g; Saturated Fat: 0g; Carbohydrates: 25g; Fiber: 3g; Sugar: 20g; Sodium: 40mg

Tips and Variations:

- Add a handful of spinach for extra nutrients without affecting the flavor.
- Substitute dairy-free yogurt for Greek yogurt for a vegan option.
- Garnish with a slice of mango or pineapple for a decorative touch.

Servings: 2

Prep Time: 5 minutes

Cook Time: 0 minutes

Total Time: 5 minutes

Ingredients:

- 1 ripe avocado
- 2 cups fresh spinach leaves
- 1 cup unsweetened almond milk (or other plant-based milk)
- 1 ripe banana
- 1 tbsp honey or maple syrup (optional)
- Handful of ice cubes

Instructions:

1. Place all ingredients in a blender.
2. Blend until smooth and creamy.
3. Taste and adjust sweetness if needed.
4. Serve immediately.
5. Enjoy!

Nutritional Information (approximate): Calories per serving: 200; Protein: 3g; Fat: 12g; Saturated Fat: 2g; Carbohydrates: 22g; Fiber: 7g; Sugar: 10g; Sodium: 80mg

Tips and Variations:

- Add a scoop of protein powder for an extra protein boost.
- Substitute spinach with kale or Swiss chard for variation.
- Top with a sprinkle of chia seeds or shredded coconut for added texture.

Chia Seed Lemonade

Servings: 2

Prep Time: 5 minutes

Cook Time: 0 minutes

Total Time: 5 minutes

Ingredients:

- 2 cups water
- 2 tbsp chia seeds
- Juice of 2 lemons
- 2 tbsp honey or maple syrup
- Handful of ice cubes

Instructions:

1. In a pitcher, combine water and chia seeds.
2. Stir well and let it sit for a few minutes to allow the chia seeds to swell.
3. Add lemon juice and honey or maple syrup.
4. Stir until sweetener is dissolved.
5. Serve over ice.
6. Enjoy!

Nutritional Information (approximate): Calories per serving: 60; Protein: 2g; Fat: 2g; Saturated Fat: 0g; Carbohydrates: 12g; Fiber: 5g; Sugar: 6g; Sodium: 10mg

Tips and Variations:

- Add a few slices of fresh ginger for a spicy kick.
- Garnish with lemon slices and fresh mint leaves for a decorative touch.
- Experiment with different citrus fruits like lime or orange for variation.

Apple Cinnamon Smoothie

Servings: 2
Prep Time: 5 minutes
Cook Time: 0 minutes
Total Time: 5 minutes

Ingredients:

- 2 apples, cored and chopped
- 1 ripe banana
- 1 cup unsweetened almond milk (or other plant-based milk)
- 1/2 tsp ground cinnamon
- 1 tbsp honey or maple syrup (optional)
- Handful of ice cubes

Instructions:

1. Place all ingredients in a blender.
2. Blend until smooth and creamy.
3. Taste and adjust sweetness if needed.
4. Serve immediately.
5. Enjoy!

Nutritional Information (approximate): Calories per serving: 130; Protein: 1g; Fat: 1g; Saturated Fat: 0g; Carbohydrates: 32g; Fiber: 5g; Sugar: 22g; Sodium: 80mg

Tips and Variations:

- Add a sprinkle of nutmeg or cloves for extra warmth.
- Use frozen banana for a thicker, creamier smoothie.
- Substitute almond milk with apple juice for a sweeter flavor.

Servings: 2

Prep Time: 5 minutes

Cook Time: 0 minutes

Total Time: 5 minutes

Ingredients:

- 1 small beetroot, peeled and chopped
- 1 cup mixed berries (such as strawberries, raspberries, blueberries)
- 1 ripe banana
- 1 cup coconut water or water
- 1 tbsp honey or maple syrup (optional)
- Handful of ice cubes

Instructions:

1. Place all ingredients in a blender.
2. Blend until smooth and creamy.
3. Taste and adjust sweetness if needed.
4. Serve immediately.
5. Enjoy!

Nutritional Information (approximate): Calories per serving: 120; Protein: 2g; Fat: 0.5g; Saturated Fat: 0g; Carbohydrates: 28g; Fiber: 5g; Sugar: 20g; Sodium: 60mg

Tips and Variations:

- Add a squeeze of fresh lemon juice for a tangy twist.
- Use frozen berries for a colder, thicker smoothie.
- Garnish with a few fresh berries or a sprig of mint for a decorative touch.

Cucumber Mint Cooler

Servings: 2

Prep Time: 5 minutes

Cook Time: 0 minutes

Total Time: 5 minutes

Ingredients:

- 1 cucumber, peeled and chopped
- Handful of fresh mint leaves
- Juice of 1 lime
- 2 cups coconut water or water
- 1 tbsp honey or maple syrup (optional)
- Handful of ice cubes

Instructions:

1. Place cucumber, mint leaves, lime juice, coconut water or water, and honey or maple syrup (if using) in a blender.
2. Blend until smooth.
3. Taste and adjust sweetness if needed.

4. Serve over ice.

5. Enjoy!

Nutritional Information (approximate): Calories per serving: 40; Protein: 1g; Fat: 0g; Saturated Fat: 0g; Carbohydrates: 10g; Fiber: 1g; Sugar: 7g; Sodium: 25mg

Tips and Variations:

- Add a pinch of salt for a savory twist.
- Substitute honey or maple syrup with stevia for a sugar-free option.
- Garnish with cucumber slices and mint leaves for a refreshing presentation.

Papaya Ginger Smoothie

Servings: 2
Prep Time: 5 minutes
Cook Time: 0 minutes
Total Time: 5 minutes

Ingredients:

- 1 ripe papaya, peeled, seeded, and chopped
- 1-inch piece of ginger, peeled
- 1 cup coconut water or water
- Juice of 1 lime
- 1 tbsp honey or maple syrup (optional)

- Handful of ice cubes

Instructions:

1. Place papaya, ginger, coconut water or water, lime juice, and honey or maple syrup (if using) in a blender.

2. Blend until smooth.

3. Taste and adjust sweetness if needed.

4. Serve over ice.

5. Enjoy!

Nutritional Information (approximate): Calories per serving: 80; Protein: 1g; Fat: 0g; Saturated Fat: 0g; Carbohydrates: 20g; Fiber: 3g; Sugar: 14g; Sodium: 25mg

Tips and Variations:

- Add a squeeze of lemon or orange juice for extra brightness.
- Include a pinch of cayenne pepper for a spicy kick.
- Garnish with a slice of lime or a sprig of mint for a decorative touch.

Servings: 2

Prep Time: 5 minutes

Cook Time: 0 minutes

Total Time: 5 minutes

Ingredients:

- 2 cups diced watermelon
- Handful of fresh basil leaves
- Juice of 1 lime
- 1-2 tbsp honey or maple syrup (optional)
- Handful of ice cubes

Instructions:

1. Place watermelon, basil leaves, lime juice, and honey or maple syrup (if using) in a blender.
2. Blend until smooth.
3. Taste and adjust sweetness if needed.
4. Serve over ice.
5. Enjoy!

Nutritional Information (approximate): Calories per serving: 50; Protein: 1g; Fat: 0g; Saturated Fat: 0g; Carbohydrates: 14g; Fiber: 1g; Sugar: 11g; Sodium: 2mg

Tips and Variations:

- Add a splash of coconut water for extra hydration.

- Garnish with a basil leaf or a slice of watermelon for a decorative touch.

- Freeze leftover watermelon in ice cube trays for future smoothies.

GLUTEN-FREE OPTIONS

Quinoa and Black Bean Salad

Servings: 4

Prep Time: 15 minutes

Cook Time: 15 minutes

Total Time: 30 minutes

Ingredients:

- 1 cup quinoa, rinsed
- 2 cups water or vegetable broth
- 1 can black beans, drained and rinsed
- 1 red bell pepper, diced
- 1/2 red onion, finely chopped
- 1 cup cherry tomatoes, halved
- 1/4 cup fresh cilantro, chopped
- Juice of 1 lime
- 2 tbsp olive oil
- Salt and pepper to taste
- Optional toppings: avocado slices, crumbled feta cheese

Instructions:

1. In a medium saucepan, combine quinoa and water or vegetable broth. Bring to a boil, then reduce heat to low, cover, and simmer for 15 minutes, or until quinoa is cooked and water is absorbed. Remove from heat and let it cool.

2. In a large bowl, combine cooked quinoa, black beans, diced red bell pepper, chopped red onion, cherry tomatoes, and chopped cilantro.

3. In a small bowl, whisk together lime juice, olive oil, salt, and pepper.

4. Pour the dressing over the salad and toss to combine.

5. Taste and adjust seasoning if needed.

6. Serve chilled or at room temperature, topped with avocado slices and crumbled feta cheese if desired.

7. Enjoy!

Nutritional Information (approximate): Calories per serving: 300; Protein: 10g; Fat: 7g; Saturated Fat: 1g; Carbohydrates: 50g; Fiber: 10g; Sugar: 3g; Sodium: 250mg

Tips and Variations:

- Add diced cucumber or avocado for extra freshness.
- Mix in some cooked corn kernels for added sweetness and texture.
- Serve as a side dish or as a main course for a vegetarian meal.

Servings: 4

Prep Time: 10 minutes

Cook Time: 15 minutes

Total Time: 25 minutes

Ingredients:

- 1 head cauliflower, riced
- 2 tbsp olive oil
- 2 cloves garlic, minced
- 1 onion, diced
- 1 bell pepper, sliced
- 1 cup broccoli florets
- 1 carrot, julienned
- 1 cup snap peas
- 2 eggs, beaten (optional)
- 3 tbsp soy sauce or tamari
- 1 tbsp sesame oil
- 2 green onions, chopped (for garnish)
- Sesame seeds (for garnish)

Instructions:

1. Heat 1 tablespoon of olive oil in a large skillet or wok over medium heat. Add minced garlic and diced onion, and cook until fragrant and onions are translucent.

2. Add sliced bell pepper, broccoli florets, julienned carrot, and snap peas to the skillet. Cook for 5-7 minutes, or until vegetables are tender-crisp.

3. Push the vegetables to one side of the skillet, and add the remaining tablespoon of olive oil to the empty side. Pour beaten eggs into the skillet and scramble until cooked through.

4. Mix the scrambled eggs with the vegetables in the skillet.

5. Stir in cauliflower rice, soy sauce or tamari, and sesame oil. Cook for another 3-5 minutes, stirring frequently, until cauliflower rice is heated through.

6. Remove from heat and garnish with chopped green onions and sesame seeds.

7. Serve hot.

8. Enjoy!

Nutritional Information (approximate): Calories per serving: 150; Protein: 6g; Fat: 8g; Saturated Fat: 1g; Carbohydrates: 15g; Fiber: 6g; Sugar: 6g; Sodium: 500mg

Tips and Variations:

- Add diced tofu, chicken, or shrimp for extra protein.
- Customize with your favorite vegetables such as mushrooms, zucchini, or snow peas.
- Use low-sodium soy sauce or tamari to reduce sodium content.

Servings: 4

Prep Time: 15 minutes

Cook Time: 40 minutes

Total Time: 55 minutes

Ingredients:

- 4 bell peppers (any color), halved and seeds removed
- 1 cup quinoa, cooked
- 1 can black beans, drained and rinsed
- 1 cup corn kernels (fresh, frozen, or canned)
- 1 cup diced tomatoes
- 1/2 cup diced onion
- 2 cloves garlic, minced
- 1 tsp ground cumin
- 1 tsp chili powder
- Salt and pepper to taste
- 1 cup shredded cheddar cheese (optional)
- Fresh cilantro, chopped (for garnish)

Instructions:

1. Preheat oven to 375°F (190°C). Grease a baking dish.
2. In a large mixing bowl, combine cooked quinoa, black beans, corn kernels, diced tomatoes, diced onion, minced garlic, ground cumin, chili powder, salt, and pepper. Mix well.

3. Stuff each bell pepper half with the quinoa mixture.

4. Place stuffed bell peppers in the prepared baking dish. If desired, sprinkle shredded cheddar cheese on top of each stuffed pepper.

5. Cover the baking dish with aluminum foil and bake in the preheated oven for 30-35 minutes, or until the peppers are tender.

6. Remove the foil and bake for an additional 5-10 minutes, or until the cheese is melted and bubbly.

7. Remove from the oven and let the stuffed peppers cool for a few minutes.

8. Garnish with chopped fresh cilantro before serving.

9. Enjoy!

Nutritional Information (approximate): Calories per serving: 250; Protein: 10g; Fat: 5g; Saturated Fat: 2g; Carbohydrates: 45g; Fiber: 10g; Sugar: 6g; Sodium: 350mg

Tips and Variations:

- Substitute quinoa with cooked rice or couscous for variation.
- Customize the filling with your favorite vegetables and spices.
- Serve with a dollop of sour cream or Greek yogurt on top.

Servings: 4
Prep Time: 10 minutes
Cook Time: 15 minutes
Total Time: 25 minutes

Ingredients:

- 4 salmon fillets
- 1 bunch asparagus, trimmed
- 2 tbsp olive oil
- 2 cloves garlic, minced
- 1 lemon, sliced
- Salt and pepper to taste
- Fresh parsley, chopped (for garnish)

Instructions:

1. Preheat oven to 400°F (200°C). Line a baking sheet with parchment paper.
2. Place salmon fillets and trimmed asparagus on the prepared baking sheet.
3. Drizzle olive oil over the salmon and asparagus. Sprinkle minced garlic evenly over the salmon.
4. Season salmon and asparagus with salt and pepper to taste.
5. Place sliced lemon rounds on top of the salmon fillets.
6. Bake in the preheated oven for 12-15 minutes, or until the salmon is cooked through and flakes easily with a fork.

7. Remove from the oven and garnish with chopped fresh parsley.

8. Serve hot.

9. Enjoy!

Nutritional Information (approximate): Calories per serving: 300; Protein: 30g; Fat: 18g; Saturated Fat: 3g; Carbohydrates: 6g; Fiber: 3g; Sugar: 2g; Sodium: 100mg

Tips and Variations:
- Add a sprinkle of dried herbs like thyme or dill for extra flavor.
- Drizzle with balsamic glaze or homemade pesto before serving.
- Serve with a side of quinoa, rice, or roasted potatoes.

Servings: 6

Prep Time: 15 minutes

Cook Time: 30 minutes

Total Time: 45 minutes

Ingredients:

- 1 cup dried lentils, rinsed
- 6 cups vegetable broth
- 2 carrots, diced
- 2 celery stalks, diced
- 1 onion, diced
- 2 cloves garlic, minced
- 1 can diced tomatoes
- 2 cups chopped kale or spinach
- 1 tsp dried thyme
- 1 tsp dried oregano
- Salt and pepper to taste
- Fresh parsley, chopped (for garnish)

Instructions:

1. In a large pot, combine dried lentils and vegetable broth. Bring to a boil, then reduce heat to low, cover, and simmer for 15 minutes.
2. Add diced carrots, celery, onion, and minced garlic to the pot. Stir to combine.

3. Continue to simmer for another 10-15 minutes, or until lentils and vegetables are tender.

4. Stir in diced tomatoes, chopped kale or spinach, dried thyme, and dried oregano.

5. Season with salt and pepper to taste.

6. Simmer for an additional 5-10 minutes to allow flavors to meld together.

7. Remove from heat and ladle into bowls.

8. Garnish with chopped fresh parsley before serving.

9. Enjoy!

Nutritional Information (approximate): Calories per serving: 200; Protein: 12g; Fat: 1g; Saturated Fat: 0g; Carbohydrates: 38g; Fiber: 12g; Sugar: 6g; Sodium: 800mg

Tips and Variations:
- Add diced potatoes or sweet potatoes for extra heartiness.
- Stir in a spoonful of miso paste for depth of flavor.
- Serve with crusty bread or a side salad for a complete meal.

Servings: 4

Prep Time: 20 minutes

Cook Time: 20 minutes

Total Time: 40 minutes

Ingredients:

- 4 boneless, skinless chicken breasts
- 1 cup quinoa, rinsed
- 2 cups water or chicken broth
- 2 cups mixed vegetables (such as bell peppers, zucchini, and broccoli), chopped
- 2 tbsp olive oil
- 2 cloves garlic, minced
- 1 tsp dried Italian seasoning
- Salt and pepper to taste
- Lemon wedges (for garnish)
- Fresh parsley, chopped (for garnish)

Instructions:

1. Preheat grill to medium-high heat.
2. Season chicken breasts with salt, pepper, and dried Italian seasoning.
3. Grill chicken breasts for 6-8 minutes per side, or until cooked through and no longer pink in the center. Remove from the grill and let them rest for a few minutes before slicing.

4. While the chicken is grilling, prepare quinoa according to package instructions. Fluff with a fork and set aside.

5. Heat olive oil in a large skillet over medium heat. Add minced garlic and sauté for 1-2 minutes, or until fragrant.

6. Add chopped mixed vegetables to the skillet and sauté for 5-7 minutes, or until tender-crisp.

7. Season vegetables with salt and pepper to taste.

8. Serve grilled chicken slices over cooked quinoa, with sautéed vegetables on the side.

9. Garnish with lemon wedges and chopped fresh parsley.

10. Enjoy!

Nutritional Information (approximate): Calories per serving: 350; Protein: 30g; Fat: 12g; Saturated Fat: 2g; Carbohydrates: 30g; Fiber: 5g; Sugar: 2g; Sodium: 300mg

Tips and Variations:
- Marinate chicken breasts in your favorite marinade for extra flavor.
- Use any combination of vegetables you prefer or have on hand.
- Drizzle balsamic glaze or pesto over the chicken and quinoa for added richness.

Servings: 4
Prep Time: 10 minutes
Cook Time: 20 minutes
Total Time: 30 minutes

Ingredients:

- 8 large eggs
- 1 cup fresh spinach leaves, chopped
- 1 cup mushrooms, sliced
- 1/2 onion, diced
- 2 cloves garlic, minced
- 1/2 cup shredded mozzarella cheese
- 2 tbsp olive oil
- Salt and pepper to taste
- Fresh parsley, chopped (for garnish)

Instructions:

1. Preheat oven to 350°F (175°C).
2. In a large bowl, whisk together eggs until well beaten. Season with salt and pepper to taste.
3. Heat olive oil in an ovenproof skillet over medium heat. Add diced onion and minced garlic, and sauté until softened and fragrant.
4. Add sliced mushrooms to the skillet and cook until they release their moisture and start to brown.

5. Stir in chopped spinach leaves and cook until wilted.

6. Pour beaten eggs into the skillet, making sure they cover the vegetables evenly.

7. Cook for 3-4 minutes, or until the edges are set.

8. Sprinkle shredded mozzarella cheese evenly over the frittata.

9. Transfer the skillet to the preheated oven and bake for 10-12 minutes, or until the frittata is set in the center and the cheese is melted and bubbly.

10. Remove from the oven and let it cool for a few minutes before slicing.

11. Garnish with chopped fresh parsley.

12. Serve hot or at room temperature.

13. Enjoy!

Nutritional Information (approximate): Calories per serving: 250; Protein: 18g; Fat: 18g; Saturated Fat: 6g; Carbohydrates: 5g; Fiber: 2g; Sugar: 2g; Sodium: 350mg

Tips and Variations:

- Add diced bell peppers or tomatoes for extra color and flavor.
- Substitute other types of cheese such as feta or goat cheese for a different taste.
- Serve with a side salad or roasted potatoes for a complete meal.

Servings: 4
Prep Time: 15 minutes
Cook Time: 10 minutes
Total Time: 25 minutes

Ingredients:

- 1 lb. shrimp, peeled and deveined
- 4 medium zucchinis, spiralized into zoodles
- 1 bell pepper, sliced
- 1 cup snap peas
- 1 carrot, julienned
- 2 cloves garlic, minced
- 2 tbsp soy sauce or tamari
- 1 tbsp sesame oil
- 1 tbsp rice vinegar
- 1 tsp honey or maple syrup (optional)
- 1 tsp grated ginger
- 2 green onions, chopped (for garnish)
- Sesame seeds (for garnish)
- Olive oil for cooking

Instructions:

1. Heat olive oil in a large skillet or wok over medium-high heat.
2. Add minced garlic and grated ginger to the skillet, and cook until fragrant.

3. Add sliced bell pepper, snap peas, and julienned carrot to the skillet. Stir-fry for 2-3 minutes, or until vegetables are tender-crisp.

4. Push the vegetables to one side of the skillet, and add shrimp to the empty side. Cook shrimp for 2-3 minutes on each side, or until pink and cooked through.

5. In a small bowl, whisk together soy sauce or tamari, sesame oil, rice vinegar, and honey or maple syrup (if using).

6. Add spiralized zucchini to the skillet, and pour the sauce over the shrimp and vegetables. Stir-fry for another 1-2 minutes, or until zoodles are heated through and coated in the sauce.

7. Remove from heat and garnish with chopped green onions and sesame seeds.

8. Serve hot.

9. Enjoy!

Nutritional Information (approximate): Calories per serving: 200; Protein: 25g; Fat: 7g; Saturated Fat: 1g; Carbohydrates: 10g; Fiber: 3g; Sugar: 6g; Sodium: 500mg

Tips and Variations:
- Add chopped broccoli or snow peas for extra crunch and nutrition.
- Customize the sauce with your favorite seasonings such as chili flakes or garlic powder.
- Serve over cooked rice or quinoa for a heartier meal.

Servings: 4
Prep Time: 15 minutes
Cook Time: 25 minutes
Total Time: 40 minutes

Ingredients:

- 1 medium butternut squash, peeled, seeded, and diced
- 2 tbsp olive oil
- 1 tsp ground cinnamon
- 1/2 tsp ground nutmeg
- Salt and pepper to taste
- 6 cups mixed salad greens
- 1/2 cup dried cranberries
- 1/4 cup crumbled feta cheese (optional)
- 1/4 cup chopped walnuts
- Balsamic vinaigrette (for dressing)

Instructions:

1. Preheat oven to 400°F (200°C). Line a baking sheet with parchment paper.
2. In a large bowl, toss diced butternut squash with olive oil, ground cinnamon, ground nutmeg, salt, and pepper until evenly coated.
3. Spread seasoned butternut squash in a single layer on the prepared baking sheet.

4. Roast in the preheated oven for 20-25 minutes, or until squash is tender and caramelized, stirring halfway through.

5. In a large salad bowl, combine mixed salad greens, dried cranberries, crumbled feta cheese (if using), and chopped walnuts.

6. Add roasted butternut squash to the salad bowl.

7. Drizzle with balsamic vinaigrette and toss to combine.

8. Serve immediately.

9. Enjoy!

Nutritional Information (approximate): Calories per serving: 200; Protein: 3g; Fat: 10g; Saturated Fat: 2g; Carbohydrates: 30g; Fiber: 6g; Sugar: 12g; Sodium: 200mg

Tips and Variations:

- Substitute dried cranberries with raisins or chopped dried apricots for a different flavor.
- Use goat cheese or blue cheese instead of feta for a tangier taste.
- Add cooked quinoa or farro for extra protein and fiber.

Servings: 4
Prep Time: 15 minutes
Cook Time: 15 minutes
Total Time: 30 minutes

Ingredients:

- 1 lb. ground chicken or turkey
- 2 tbsp olive oil
- 1 onion, diced
- 2 cloves garlic, minced
- 1 red bell pepper, diced
- 1 cup mushrooms, chopped
- 1/4 cup hoisin sauce
- 2 tbsp soy sauce or tamari
- 1 tbsp rice vinegar
- 1 tsp sesame oil
- 1 tsp grated ginger
- 1/4 cup chopped green onions
- Salt and pepper to taste
- Butter lettuce leaves (for serving)
- Optional toppings: chopped peanuts, sliced green onions, chopped cilantro, sriracha sauce

Instructions:

1. Heat olive oil in a large skillet over medium-high heat.
2. Add diced onion and minced garlic to the skillet, and sauté until softened and fragrant.
3. Add ground chicken or turkey to the skillet, breaking it apart with a spoon. Cook until browned and cooked through.
4. Stir in diced red bell pepper and chopped mushrooms, and cook for 2-3 minutes, or until vegetables are tender.
5. In a small bowl, whisk together hoisin sauce, soy sauce or tamari, rice vinegar, sesame oil, and grated ginger.
6. Pour the sauce over the chicken mixture in the skillet, and stir to combine. Cook for another 2-3 minutes, or until heated through.
7. Stir in chopped green onions, and season with salt and pepper to taste.
8. Remove from heat.
9. To serve, spoon the chicken mixture into butter lettuce leaves, creating wraps.
10. Garnish with chopped peanuts, sliced green onions, chopped cilantro, and sriracha sauce if desired.

Nutritional Information (approximate): Calories per serving: 250; Protein: 20g; Fat: 15g; Saturated Fat: 3g; Carbohydrates: 10g; Fiber: 2g; Sugar: 6g; Sodium: 600mg

Tips and Variations:

- Substitute ground chicken or turkey with tofu or tempeh for a vegetarian option.
- Add diced water chestnuts or bamboo shoots for extra crunch.

Servings: 4

Prep Time: 15 minutes

Cook Time: 25 minutes

Total Time: 40 minutes

Ingredients:

- 1 lb. boneless, skinless chicken breasts or thighs, cut into bite-sized pieces
- 2 tbsp olive oil
- 1 onion, diced
- 2 cloves garlic, minced
- 1 red bell pepper, sliced
- 1 cup broccoli florets
- 1 carrot, sliced
- 1 can (13.5 oz) coconut milk
- 2 tbsp red curry paste
- 1 tbsp soy sauce or tamari
- 1 tbsp maple syrup or honey
- 1 tbsp lime juice
- Salt and pepper to taste
- Fresh cilantro, chopped (for garnish)
- Cooked rice or quinoa (for serving)

Instructions:

1. Heat olive oil in a large skillet or wok over medium-high heat.
2. Add diced onion and minced garlic to the skillet, and sauté until softened and fragrant.

3. Add chicken pieces to the skillet, and cook until browned on all sides.

4. Stir in sliced red bell pepper, broccoli florets, and sliced carrot. Cook for 3-4 minutes, or until vegetables are tender-crisp.

5. In a small bowl, whisk together coconut milk, red curry paste, soy sauce or tamari, maple syrup or honey, lime juice, salt, and pepper.

6. Pour the curry sauce over the chicken and vegetables in the skillet, and stir to combine.

7. Bring to a simmer, then reduce heat to low and let it simmer for 10-15 minutes, or until chicken is cooked through and flavors have melded together.

8. Taste and adjust seasoning if needed.

9. Remove from heat.

10. Serve hot over cooked rice or quinoa, garnished with chopped fresh cilantro.

11. Enjoy!

Nutritional Information (approximate): Calories per serving: 350; Protein: 25g; Fat: 20g; Saturated Fat: 12g; Carbohydrates: 15g; Fiber: 3g; Sugar: 6g; Sodium: 500mg

Tips and Variations:

- Customize the vegetables with your favorites such as snow peas, bell peppers, or spinach.
- Use green curry paste for a different flavor profile.
- Garnish with sliced red chili peppers or crushed peanuts for extra heat and crunch.

Servings: 4

Prep Time: 15 minutes

Cook Time: 0 minutes

Total Time: 15 minutes

Ingredients:

- 2 cans (15 oz each) chickpeas, drained and rinsed
- 1 cucumber, diced
- 1 bell pepper (any color), diced
- 1 cup cherry tomatoes, halved
- 1/2 red onion, thinly sliced
- 1/4 cup Kalamata olives, pitted and halved
- 1/4 cup crumbled feta cheese
- 2 tbsp chopped fresh parsley
- 2 tbsp chopped fresh basil
- 2 tbsp olive oil
- 1 tbsp red wine vinegar
- 1 tsp dried oregano
- Salt and pepper to taste
- Lemon wedges (for serving)

Instructions:

1. In a large mixing bowl, combine drained and rinsed chickpeas, diced cucumber, diced bell pepper, halved cherry tomatoes, thinly sliced red

onion, halved Kalamata olives, crumbled feta cheese, chopped fresh parsley, and chopped fresh basil.

2. In a small bowl, whisk together olive oil, red wine vinegar, dried oregano, salt, and pepper.
3. Pour the dressing over the chickpea salad, and toss gently to combine.
4. Taste and adjust seasoning if needed.
5. Serve the salad at room temperature or chilled, with lemon wedges on the side.
6. Enjoy!

Nutritional Information (approximate): Calories per serving: 300; Protein: 12g; Fat: 10g; Saturated Fat: 2g; Carbohydrates: 25g; Fiber: 8g; Sugar: 6g; Sodium: 600mg

Tips and Variations:
- Add diced avocado or artichoke hearts for extra creaminess and flavor.
- Customize with your favorite Mediterranean ingredients such as roasted red peppers or sun-dried tomatoes.
- Serve as a side dish or as a light main course for lunch.

VEGAN AND VEGETARIAN VARIATIONS

Servings: 4
Prep Time: 10 minutes
Cook Time: 0 minutes
Total Time: 10 minutes

Ingredients:

- 2 cans (15 oz each) chickpeas, drained and rinsed
- 1 large avocado, diced
- 1 cucumber, diced
- 1 bell pepper (any color), diced
- 1/4 red onion, thinly sliced
- 1/4 cup chopped fresh parsley
- 2 tbsp olive oil
- 2 tbsp lemon juice
- Salt and pepper to taste

Instructions:

1. In a large mixing bowl, combine chickpeas, diced avocado, diced cucumber, diced bell pepper, thinly sliced red onion, and chopped fresh parsley.
2. Drizzle olive oil and lemon juice over the salad.
3. Season with salt and pepper to taste.
4. Toss gently until all ingredients are evenly coated with the dressing.

5. Serve immediately or refrigerate until ready to serve.

6. Enjoy!

Nutritional Information (approximate): Calories per serving: 300; Protein: 10g; Fat: 15g; Saturated Fat: 2g; Carbohydrates: 35g; Fiber: 12g; Sugar: 5g; Sodium: 400mg

Tips and Variations:

- Add cherry tomatoes or olives for extra flavor.
- Sprinkle with feta cheese or nutritional yeast for a different taste.
- Serve over a bed of mixed greens for a light lunch or dinner.

Quinoa Stuffed Bell Peppers

Servings: 4
Prep Time: 15 minutes
Cook Time: 30 minutes
Total Time: 45 minutes

Ingredients:

- 4 bell peppers (any color)
- 1 cup quinoa, rinsed
- 2 cups vegetable broth
- 1 can (15 oz) black beans, drained and rinsed
- 1 cup corn kernels (fresh, frozen, or canned)
- 1 cup diced tomatoes

- 1/2 cup diced red onion
- 2 cloves garlic, minced
- 1 tsp ground cumin
- 1 tsp chili powder
- Salt and pepper to taste
- 1/2 cup shredded cheddar cheese or vegan cheese (optional)
- Fresh cilantro, chopped (for garnish)

Instructions:

1. Preheat the oven to 375°F (190°C).
2. Cut the tops off the bell peppers and remove the seeds and membranes.
3. In a medium saucepan, bring vegetable broth to a boil. Add quinoa, reduce heat to low, cover, and simmer for 15-20 minutes, or until quinoa is cooked and liquid is absorbed.
4. In a large mixing bowl, combine cooked quinoa, black beans, corn kernels, diced tomatoes, diced red onion, minced garlic, ground cumin, chili powder, salt, and pepper.
5. Spoon the quinoa mixture into the hollowed-out bell peppers, pressing down gently to pack the filling.
6. Place stuffed bell peppers in a baking dish, standing upright.
7. If using cheese, sprinkle shredded cheese over the tops of the stuffed peppers.
8. Cover the baking dish with aluminum foil and bake in the preheated oven for 25-30 minutes, or until the peppers are tender.
9. Remove the foil and bake for an additional 5 minutes, or until the cheese is melted and bubbly.

10. Remove from the oven and let them cool for a few minutes before serving.

11. Garnish with chopped fresh cilantro.

12. Enjoy!

Nutritional Information (approximate): Calories per serving: 350; Protein: 15g; Fat: 8g; Saturated Fat: 3g; Carbohydrates: 55g; Fiber: 12g; Sugar: 8g; Sodium: 600mg

Tips and Variations:
- Use different colored bell peppers for a visually appealing presentation.
- Substitute quinoa with cooked rice or couscous if desired.
- Customize the filling with your favorite vegetables and spices.

Servings: 4
Prep Time: 10 minutes
Cook Time: 30 minutes
Total Time: 40 minutes

Ingredients:

- 1 cup dried green lentils, rinsed
- 4 cups vegetable broth
- 1 onion, diced
- 2 cloves garlic, minced
- 2 carrots, diced
- 2 celery stalks, diced
- 1 can (14 oz) diced tomatoes
- 2 cups chopped spinach
- 1 tsp ground cumin
- 1 tsp paprika
- Salt and pepper to taste
- Olive oil for cooking
- Fresh parsley, chopped (for garnish)

Instructions:

1. In a large pot, heat olive oil over medium heat.
2. Add diced onion and minced garlic to the pot, and sauté until softened and fragrant.

3. Stir in diced carrots and diced celery, and cook for 3-4 minutes, or until slightly softened.
4. Add dried green lentils, vegetable broth, diced tomatoes (with their juices), ground cumin, paprika, salt, and pepper to the pot. Stir to combine.
5. Bring the stew to a boil, then reduce heat to low, cover, and simmer for 20-25 minutes, or until lentils are tender.
6. Stir in chopped spinach and cook for an additional 2-3 minutes, or until spinach is wilted.
7. Taste and adjust seasoning if needed.
8. Remove from heat and let it cool for a few minutes before serving.
9. Ladle the stew into bowls, garnish with chopped fresh parsley, and serve hot. Enjoy!

Nutritional Information (approximate): Calories per serving: 250; Protein: 15g; Fat: 2g; Saturated Fat: 0g; Carbohydrates: 45g; Fiber: 15g; Sugar: 8g; Sodium: 700mg

Tips and Variations:
- Add other vegetables such as bell peppers or zucchini for extra flavor and nutrients.
- Stir in a tablespoon of balsamic vinegar for added depth of flavor.
- Serve the stew over cooked quinoa or brown rice for a complete meal.

Servings: 4
Prep Time: 10 minutes
Cook Time: 20 minutes
Total Time: 30 minutes

Ingredients:

- 8 oz (225g) fettuccine or any pasta of your choice
- 2 tbsp olive oil
- 1 onion, diced
- 2 cloves garlic, minced
- 8 oz (225g) mushrooms, sliced
- 1 can (14 oz) coconut milk
- 2 tbsp soy sauce or tamari
- 1 tbsp Dijon mustard
- 1 tsp smoked paprika
- Salt and pepper to taste
- Fresh parsley, chopped (for garnish)

Instructions:

1. Cook the pasta according to the package instructions until al dente. Drain and set aside.
2. In a large skillet, heat olive oil over medium heat.
3. Add diced onion and minced garlic to the skillet, and sauté until softened and fragrant.

4. Add sliced mushrooms to the skillet, and cook until they release their moisture and start to brown.

5. Stir in coconut milk, soy sauce or tamari, Dijon mustard, and smoked paprika. Bring to a simmer.

6. Let the sauce simmer for 5-7 minutes, or until slightly thickened.

7. Season with salt and pepper to taste.

8. Add cooked pasta to the skillet, and toss to coat evenly with the sauce.

9. Cook for another 2-3 minutes, or until heated through.

10. Remove from heat and let it cool for a few minutes before serving.

11. Garnish with chopped fresh parsley.

12. Serve hot.

13. Enjoy!

Nutritional Information (approximate): Calories per serving: 400; Protein: 10g; Fat: 20g; Saturated Fat: 12g; Carbohydrates: 45g; Fiber: 5g; Sugar: 3g; Sodium: 500mg

Tips and Variations:
- Use vegetable broth instead of coconut milk for a lighter version of the sauce.
- Add a splash of white wine or vegetable broth for extra flavor.
- Serve with a side of steamed vegetables or a green salad for a balanced meal.

Servings: 4

Prep Time: 10 minutes

Cook Time: 10 minutes

Total Time: 20 minutes

Ingredients:

- 4 medium zucchini, spiralized into noodles
- 2 tbsp olive oil
- 2 cloves garlic, minced
- 1 can (14 oz) diced tomatoes
- 1/4 cup tomato paste
- 1 tsp dried oregano
- 1 tsp dried basil
- Salt and pepper to taste
- Fresh basil leaves, chopped (for garnish)
- Vegan parmesan cheese (optional)

Instructions:

1. Heat olive oil in a large skillet over medium heat.
2. Add minced garlic to the skillet, and sauté until fragrant.
3. Add diced tomatoes, tomato paste, dried oregano, dried basil, salt, and pepper to the skillet. Stir to combine.
4. Let the marinara sauce simmer for 5-7 minutes, or until slightly thickened.

5. While the sauce is simmering, spiralize the zucchini into noodles using a spiralizer.

6. Add zucchini noodles to the skillet, and toss to coat evenly with the marinara sauce.

7. Cook for 2-3 minutes, or until the zucchini noodles are heated through but still crisp-tender.

8. Remove from heat and let it cool for a few minutes before serving.

9. Garnish with chopped fresh basil leaves and vegan parmesan cheese if desired.

10. Serve hot.

11. Enjoy!

Nutritional Information (approximate): Calories per serving: 100; Protein: 3g; Fat: 7g; Saturated Fat: 1g; Carbohydrates: 10g; Fiber: 3g; Sugar: 6g; Sodium: 300mg

Tips and Variations:

- Add diced onions or bell peppers to the sauce for extra flavor and texture.
- Top with pine nuts or toasted breadcrumbs for added crunch.
- Serve with a side of garlic bread or a green salad for a complete meal.

Servings: 4

Prep Time: 15 minutes

Cook Time: 15 minutes

Total Time: 30 minutes

Ingredients:

- 14 oz (400g) firm tofu, pressed and cubed
- 2 tbsp soy sauce or tamari
- 1 tbsp rice vinegar
- 1 tbsp maple syrup or honey
- 2 tbsp sesame oil, divided
- 1 onion, thinly sliced
- 2 cloves garlic, minced
- 1 bell pepper (any color), thinly sliced
- 1 cup broccoli florets
- 1 cup snap peas
- 1 carrot, julienned
- 2 green onions, chopped
- Sesame seeds (for garnish

Instructions:

1. In a small bowl, whisk together soy sauce or tamari, rice vinegar, maple syrup or honey, and 1 tablespoon of sesame oil.

2. Place the cubed tofu in a shallow dish and pour the marinade over it. Let it marinate for at least 10 minutes.

3. Heat the remaining tablespoon of sesame oil in a large skillet or wok over medium-high heat.

4. Add the marinated tofu to the skillet and cook until golden brown on all sides. Remove from the skillet and set aside.

5. In the same skillet, add the sliced onion and minced garlic. Stir-fry for 2-3 minutes, or until softened and fragrant.

6. Add the sliced bell pepper, broccoli florets, snap peas, and julienned carrot to the skillet. Stir-fry for an additional 3-4 minutes, or until the vegetables are tender-crisp.

7. Return the cooked tofu to the skillet and toss everything together to combine.

8. Cook for another 2-3 minutes, or until heated through.

9. Remove from heat and garnish with chopped green onions and sesame seeds.

10. Serve hot over cooked rice or noodles. Enjoy!

Nutritional Information (approximate): Calories per serving: 250; Protein: 15g; Fat: 15g; Saturated Fat: 2g; Carbohydrates: 20g; Fiber: 5g; Sugar: 8g; Sodium: 600mg

Tips and Variations:

- Add other vegetables like mushrooms, baby corn, or water chestnuts for extra variety.
- For a spicy kick, add some sriracha or chili flakes to the stir-fry sauce.
- Garnish with fresh cilantro or chopped peanuts for added flavor and texture.

Servings: 4

Prep Time: 15 minutes

Cook Time: 25 minutes

Total Time: 40 minutes

Ingredients:

For the falafel:

- 1 can (15 oz) chickpeas, drained and rinsed
- 1/4 cup chopped fresh parsley
- 1/4 cup chopped fresh cilantro
- 1/4 cup diced red onion
- 2 cloves garlic, minced
- 1 tsp ground cumin
- 1 tsp ground coriander
- 1/2 tsp baking powder
- Salt and pepper to taste
- 2 tbsp olive oil

For the tahini sauce:

- 1/4 cup tahini
- 2 tbsp lemon juice
- 2 tbsp water
- 1 clove garlic, minced
- Salt to taste

Instructions:

For the falafel:

1. Preheat the oven to 375°F (190°C). Line a baking sheet with parchment paper.
2. In a food processor, combine chickpeas, chopped fresh parsley, chopped fresh cilantro, diced red onion, minced garlic, ground cumin, ground coriander, baking powder, salt, and pepper.
3. Pulse until the mixture is well combined but still slightly chunky.
4. Form the mixture into small balls or patties and place them on the prepared baking sheet.
5. Brush the falafel with olive oil.
6. Bake in the preheated oven for 20-25 minutes, or until golden brown and crispy, flipping halfway through.

For the tahini sauce:

1. In a small bowl, whisk together tahini, lemon juice, water, minced garlic, and salt until smooth.
2. If the sauce is too thick, add more water until desired consistency is reached.

To serve:

1. Serve the baked falafel hot out of the oven with the tahini sauce drizzled on top.
2. Enjoy!

Nutritional Information (approximate): Calories per serving: 250; Protein: 8g; Fat: 15g; Saturated Fat: 2g; Carbohydrates: 25g; Fiber: 6g; Sugar: 3g; Sodium: 300mg

Tips and Variations:

- For extra flavor, add a pinch of ground turmeric or smoked paprika to the falafel mixture.
- Serve the falafel with pita bread, hummus, and a side salad for a complete meal.
- Leftover falafel can be stored in an airtight container in the refrigerator for up to 3 days. Reheat in the oven or toaster oven before serving.

Vegan Buddha Bowl

Servings: 4
Prep Time: 15 minutes
Cook Time: 30 minutes
Total Time: 45 minutes

Ingredients:
For the roasted vegetables:

- 2 cups cauliflower florets
- 2 cups sweet potato, peeled and cubed
- 1 cup Brussels sprouts, halved
- 2 tbsp olive oil
- 1 tsp smoked paprika

- 1 tsp garlic powder
- Salt and pepper to taste

For the quinoa:
- 1 cup quinoa, rinsed
- 2 cups vegetable broth or water

For the tahini dressing:
- 1/4 cup tahini
- 2 tbsp lemon juice
- 2 tbsp water
- 1 clove garlic, minced
- Salt to taste

For assembling:
- 2 cups baby spinach or mixed greens
- 1 avocado, sliced
- 1/4 cup pumpkin seeds
- Fresh cilantro or parsley, chopped (for garnish)

Instructions:

For the roasted vegetables:

1. Preheat the oven to 400°F (200°C). Line a baking sheet with parchment paper.
2. In a large bowl, toss cauliflower florets, sweet potato cubes, and Brussels sprouts halves with olive oil, smoked paprika, garlic powder, salt, and pepper until evenly coated.

3. Spread the seasoned vegetables in a single layer on the prepared baking sheet.

4. Roast in the preheated oven for 25-30 minutes, or until golden brown and tender, stirring halfway through.

For the quinoa:

1. In a medium saucepan, bring vegetable broth or water to a boil.

2. Add rinsed quinoa to the saucepan, reduce heat to low, cover, and simmer for 15-20 minutes, or until quinoa is cooked and liquid is absorbed.

3. Fluff the quinoa with a fork and set aside.

For the tahini dressing:

1. In a small bowl, whisk together tahini, lemon juice, water, minced garlic, and salt until smooth.

2. If the dressing is too thick, add more water until desired consistency is reached.

To assemble:

1. Divide cooked quinoa, roasted vegetables, baby spinach or mixed greens, and sliced avocado among serving bowls.

2. Drizzle tahini dressing over each bowl.

3. Sprinkle pumpkin seeds and chopped fresh cilantro or parsley on top for garnish.

4. Serve immediately and enjoy!

Nutritional Information (approximate): Calories per serving: 400; Protein: 12g; Fat: 22g; Saturated Fat: 3g; Carbohydrates: 42g; Fiber: 10g; Sugar: 5g; Sodium: 300mg

Tips and Variations:

- Feel free to customize your Buddha bowl with your favorite vegetables and grains. Roasted chickpeas, quinoa, brown rice, or barley are great alternatives to quinoa.
- Add a squeeze of fresh lemon juice or a drizzle of balsamic glaze for extra flavor.
- For added protein, top with grilled tofu, tempeh, or a sprinkle of nutritional yeast.

Cauliflower Tacos

Servings: 4
Prep Time: 15 minutes
Cook Time: 25 minutes
Total Time: 40 minutes

Ingredients:

For the cauliflower filling:

- 1 medium head cauliflower, cut into small florets
- 2 tbsp olive oil
- 1 tsp chili powder
- 1 tsp ground cumin

- 1/2 tsp smoked paprika
- 1/2 tsp garlic powder
- Salt and pepper to taste

For the tacos:
- 8 small corn or flour tortillas
- 1 cup shredded red cabbage
- 1 avocado, sliced
- Fresh cilantro leaves
- Lime wedges
- Hot sauce or salsa (optional)

Instructions:

For the cauliflower filling:
1. Preheat the oven to 425°F (220°C). Line a baking sheet with parchment paper.
2. In a large bowl, toss cauliflower florets with olive oil, chili powder, ground cumin, smoked paprika, garlic powder, salt, and pepper until evenly coated.
3. Spread the seasoned cauliflower in a single layer on the prepared baking sheet.
4. Roast in the preheated oven for 20-25 minutes, or until the cauliflower is tender and slightly browned, stirring halfway through.

For the tacos:
1. Warm the tortillas according to package instructions.
2. Divide the roasted cauliflower filling among the tortillas.

3. Top each taco with shredded red cabbage, sliced avocado, and fresh cilantro leaves.

4. Squeeze a lime wedge over each taco and serve with hot sauce or salsa if desired.

5. Serve immediately and enjoy!

Nutritional Information (approximate): Calories per serving: 200; Protein: 5g; Fat: 8g; Saturated Fat: 1g; Carbohydrates: 30g; Fiber: 6g; Sugar: 4g; Sodium: 300mg

Tips and Variations:
- Add your favorite toppings such as diced tomatoes, jalapeños, or pickled onions.
- Serve with a side of black beans, refried beans, or Mexican rice for a complete meal.
- Use lettuce leaves or corn tortillas for a low-carb or gluten-free option.

Servings: 6

Prep Time: 15 minutes

Cook Time: 1 hour

Total Time: 1 hour 15 minutes

Ingredients:

For the lentil loaf:

- 1 cup green lentils, rinsed
- 2 1/2 cups vegetable broth or water
- 1 onion, finely chopped
- 2 cloves garlic, minced
- 1 carrot, grated
- 1 celery stalk, finely chopped
- 1/2 cup rolled oats
- 1/4 cup tomato paste
- 2 tbsp soy sauce or tamari
- 1 tbsp ground flaxseed
- 1 tsp dried thyme
- 1 tsp dried oregano
- 1/2 tsp smoked paprika
- Salt and pepper to taste

For the glaze:

- 1/4 cup ketchup
- 2 tbsp maple syrup or brown sugar

- 1 tbsp balsamic vinegar
- 1 tsp Dijon mustard

Instructions:

For the lentil loaf:

1. Preheat the oven to 375°F (190°C). Lightly grease a loaf pan and set aside.
2. In a medium saucepan, combine green lentils and vegetable broth or water. Bring to a boil, then reduce heat to low, cover, and simmer for 25-30 minutes, or until lentils are tender and liquid is absorbed.
3. In a large skillet, heat olive oil over medium heat. Add chopped onion, minced garlic, grated carrot, and chopped celery. Sauté until vegetables are softened, about 5-7 minutes.
4. In a large mixing bowl, combine cooked lentils, sautéed vegetables, rolled oats, tomato paste, soy sauce or tamari, ground flaxseed, dried thyme, dried oregano, smoked paprika, salt, and pepper. Mix until well combined.
5. Transfer the lentil mixture to the prepared loaf pan and press it down firmly.

For the glaze:

6. In a small bowl, whisk together ketchup, maple syrup or brown sugar, balsamic vinegar, and Dijon mustard until smooth.
7. Spread the glaze evenly over the top of the lentil loaf.
8. Bake in the preheated oven for 40-45 minutes, or until the loaf is firm and the glaze is caramelized.
9. Remove from the oven and let it cool for a few minutes before slicing.
10. Serve slices of lentil loaf with your favorite side dishes. Enjoy!

Nutritional Information (approximate): Calories per serving: 250; Protein: 12g; Fat: 3g; Saturated Fat: 0.5g; Carbohydrates: 45g; Fiber: 10g; Sugar: 8g; Sodium: 600mg

Tips and Variations:

- Serve the lentil loaf with mashed potatoes, gravy, and steamed vegetables for a classic comfort meal.
- Leftover slices can be refrigerated in an airtight container for up to 5 days or frozen for up to 3 months. Reheat in the microwave or oven before serving.

Roasted Veggie Power Bowl

Servings: 4
Prep Time: 15 minutes
Cook Time: 25 minutes
Total Time: 40 minutes

Ingredients:

For the roasted vegetables:

- 2 cups Brussels sprouts, halved
- 2 cups cauliflower florets
- 2 cups sweet potato, peeled and cubed
- 1 red onion, sliced
- 2 tbsp olive oil
- 1 tsp smoked paprika

- 1 tsp garlic powder
- Salt and pepper to taste

For the quinoa:

- 1 cup quinoa, rinsed
- 2 cups vegetable broth or water

For the tahini dressing:

- 1/4 cup tahini
- 2 tbsp lemon juice
- 2 tbsp water
- 1 clove garlic, minced
- Salt to taste

For assembling:

- 2 cups baby spinach or mixed greens
- 1 avocado, sliced
- 1/4 cup pumpkin seeds
- Fresh cilantro or parsley, chopped (for garnish)

Instructions:

For the roasted vegetables:

1. Preheat the oven to 425°F (220°C). Line a baking sheet with parchment paper.
2. In a large bowl, toss Brussels sprouts, cauliflower florets, sweet potato cubes, and sliced red onion with olive oil, smoked paprika, garlic powder, salt, and pepper until evenly coated.

3. Spread the seasoned vegetables in a single layer on the prepared baking sheet.

4. Roast in the preheated oven for 20-25 minutes, or until the vegetables are tender and caramelized, stirring halfway through.

For the quinoa:

1. In a medium saucepan, bring vegetable broth or water to a boil.

2. Add rinsed quinoa to the saucepan, reduce heat to low, cover, and simmer for 15-20 minutes, or until quinoa is cooked and liquid is absorbed. 3. Fluff the quinoa with a fork and set aside.

For the tahini dressing:

1. In a small bowl, whisk together tahini, lemon juice, water, minced garlic, and salt until smooth.

2. If the dressing is too thick, add more water until desired consistency is reached.

To assemble:

1. Divide cooked quinoa, roasted vegetables, baby spinach or mixed greens, and sliced avocado among serving bowls.

2. Drizzle tahini dressing over each bowl.

3. Sprinkle pumpkin seeds and chopped fresh cilantro or parsley on top for garnish.

4. Serve immediately and enjoy!

Nutritional Information (approximate): Calories per serving: 400; Protein: 12g; Fat: 20g; Saturated Fat: 3g; Carbohydrates: 45g; Fiber: 12g; Sugar: 8g; Sodium: 300mg

Tips and Variations:

- Feel free to use your favorite vegetables for roasting, such as broccoli, carrots, or bell peppers.
- Add a squeeze of fresh lemon juice or a drizzle of balsamic glaze for extra flavor.
- Top with grilled tofu, tempeh, or chickpeas for added protein.

Vegan Pumpkin Curry

Servings: 4
Prep Time: 15 minutes
Cook Time: 25 minutes
Total Time: 40 minutes

Ingredients:

- 2 cups pumpkin or butternut squash, peeled and cubed
- 1 can (14 oz) coconut milk
- 1 onion, finely chopped
- 2 cloves garlic, minced
- 1-inch piece ginger, grated
- 1 red chili, finely chopped (optional)
- 1 tbsp red curry paste

- 1 tsp ground turmeric
- 1 tsp ground cumin
- 1 tsp ground coriander
- 1 cup vegetable broth
- 1 cup baby spinach or kale
- 1 tbsp coconut oil or olive oil
- Salt and pepper to taste
- Fresh cilantro, chopped (for garnish)

Instructions:

1. In a large skillet or pot, heat coconut oil or olive oil over medium heat.
2. Add chopped onion, minced garlic, grated ginger, and chopped red chili (if using). Sauté until the onion is soft and translucent.
3. Stir in red curry paste, ground turmeric, ground cumin, and ground coriander. Cook for another minute until fragrant.
4. Add cubed pumpkin or butternut squash to the skillet and toss to coat in the spice mixture.
5. Pour in coconut milk and vegetable broth. Bring to a simmer and cook for 15-20 minutes, or until the pumpkin is tender.
6. Stir in baby spinach or kale and cook until wilted.
7. Season with salt and pepper to taste.
8. Remove from heat and garnish with chopped fresh cilantro.
9. Serve hot over cooked rice or quinoa.
10. Enjoy!

Nutritional Information (approximate): Calories per serving: 250; Protein: 5g; Fat: 20g; Saturated Fat: 15g; Carbohydrates: 20g; Fiber: 5g; Sugar: 5g; Sodium: 400mg

Tips and Variations:

- Add diced tofu, chickpeas, or lentils for extra protein.
- Garnish with a squeeze of fresh lime juice or a dollop of coconut yogurt for added freshness.
- For a spicier curry, increase the amount of red chili or add a pinch of cayenne pepper. Adjust the seasoning according to your taste preference.

Vegan Black Bean Burgers

Servings: 4
Prep Time: 15 minutes
Cook Time: 15 minutes
Total Time: 30 minutes

Ingredients:

- 1 can (15 oz) black beans, drained and rinsed
- 1/2 cup rolled oats
- 1/4 cup finely chopped onion
- 2 cloves garlic, minced
- 1/4 cup chopped fresh cilantro
- 1 tsp ground cumin
- 1/2 tsp chili powder

- Salt and pepper to taste
- 1 tbsp olive oil (for cooking)

For serving:
- Burger buns
- Lettuce leaves
- Sliced tomato
- Sliced avocado
- Red onion slices
- Ketchup, mustard, or your favorite condiments

Instructions:
1. In a large mixing bowl, mash black beans with a fork or potato masher until mostly smooth but still slightly chunky.
2. Add rolled oats, finely chopped onion, minced garlic, chopped fresh cilantro, ground cumin, chili powder, salt, and pepper to the mashed black beans. Mix until well combined.
3. Divide the mixture into 4 equal portions and shape each portion into a burger patty.
4. Heat olive oil in a skillet over medium heat.
5. Add the black bean burger patties to the skillet and cook for 5-7 minutes on each side, or until golden brown and heated through.
6. Toast the burger buns if desired.
7. Assemble the burgers by placing lettuce leaves, a black bean burger patty, sliced tomato, sliced avocado, and red onion slices on the bottom half of each bun.

8. Spread ketchup, mustard, or your favorite condiments on the top half of the bun.

9. Place the top half of the bun over the fillings to complete the burgers.

10. Serve immediately and enjoy!

Nutritional Information (approximate): Calories per serving (without bun and toppings): 150; Protein: 7g; Fat: 4g; Saturated Fat: 0.5g; Carbohydrates: 23g; Fiber: 7g; Sugar: 1g; Sodium: 250mg

Tips and Variations:

- Customize your black bean burgers with your favorite toppings and condiments. Try adding sliced pickles, jalapeños, or vegan cheese for extra flavor.
- Serve the burgers with a side of sweet potato fries, coleslaw, or a simple green salad for a complete meal.
- Leftover black bean burger patties can be refrigerated in an airtight container for up to 3 days or frozen for up to 3 months. Reheat in the oven or microwave before serving.

LIFESTYLE TIPS

Embracing an anti-inflammatory lifestyle extends beyond diet. Incorporating regular exercise, managing stress effectively, and ensuring quality sleep are crucial elements that work together to reduce inflammation and promote overall wellness. In this chapter, we will explore these three essential aspects and provide practical tips to integrate them into your daily routine.

Incorporating Exercise

Regular physical activity is a powerful tool for reducing inflammation and improving your overall health. Exercise helps regulate inflammatory markers, boosts your immune system, and enhances your mood. Here are some guidelines and tips to help you incorporate exercise into your lifestyle:

1. Choose the Right Activities

- **Aerobic Exercise**: Engage in activities like walking, jogging, swimming, or cycling for at least 150 minutes per week. These exercises help improve cardiovascular health and reduce inflammation.

- **Strength Training**: Include resistance exercises such as weight lifting, bodyweight exercises, or resistance bands at least twice a week to build muscle and support joint health.

- **Flexibility and Balance**: Incorporate activities like yoga, Pilates, or tai chi to enhance flexibility, balance, and overall well-being.

2. Start Slow and Build Gradually

- **Begin with Low-Intensity Exercises**: If you're new to exercising, start with low-impact activities like walking or gentle yoga to avoid injury and build your fitness level gradually.

- **Increase Intensity Over Time**: Gradually increase the intensity and duration of your workouts as your fitness improves. Listen to your body and avoid overexertion.

3. Make Exercise Enjoyable

- **Find Activities You Enjoy**: Choose exercises that you find fun and engaging, whether it's dancing, hiking, or playing a sport. This will make it easier to stay motivated and consistent.

- **Exercise with Others**: Join a fitness class, workout with a friend, or participate in group activities to stay motivated and make exercising a social activity.

4. Incorporate Movement into Your Daily Routine

- **Take Breaks to Move**: If you have a sedentary job, take regular breaks to stand, stretch, and walk around. Aim to move for at least a few minutes every hour.

- **Use Active Transportation**: Whenever possible, walk or bike instead of driving. Opt for stairs instead of elevators to increase your daily physical activity.

Stress Management

Chronic stress can significantly contribute to inflammation and negatively impact your health. Effectively managing stress is essential for maintaining a balanced, anti-inflammatory lifestyle. Here are some strategies to help you manage stress:

1. Practice Mindfulness and Relaxation Techniques

- **Meditation**: Spend a few minutes each day practicing mindfulness meditation to reduce stress and promote mental clarity.

- **Deep Breathing**: Practice deep breathing exercises to calm your nervous system and reduce stress levels.

- **Progressive Muscle Relaxation**: Tense and then slowly release each muscle group in your body to reduce physical tension and stress.

2. Stay Connected

- **Build Supportive Relationships**: Maintain strong connections with family and friends. Social support is crucial for managing stress and enhancing your emotional well-being.

- **Join Support Groups**: Consider joining a support group or community organization related to your interests or health conditions to share experiences and gain encouragement.

3. Engage in Hobbies and Leisure Activities

- **Pursue Interests**: Engage in activities and hobbies that you enjoy and that bring you joy, such as reading, gardening, painting, or playing a musical instrument.

- **Schedule Downtime**: Make time for relaxation and leisure in your daily routine to unwind and recharge.

4. Practice Time Management

- **Prioritize Tasks**: Focus on important tasks and set realistic goals to avoid feeling overwhelmed.

- **Delegate Responsibilities**: Share responsibilities with others to reduce your workload and manage stress more effectively.

Ensuring Quality Sleep

Quality sleep is vital for reducing inflammation and maintaining overall health. Poor sleep can lead to increased stress, weight gain, and higher levels of inflammatory markers. Here are some tips to improve your sleep hygiene:

1. Establish a Consistent Sleep Schedule

- **Regular Sleep and Wake Times**: Go to bed and wake up at the same time every day, even on weekends, to regulate your body's internal clock.

- **Create a Relaxing Bedtime Routine**: Develop a calming pre-sleep routine, such as reading a book, taking a warm bath, or practicing gentle yoga to signal to your body that it's time to wind down.

2. Optimize Your Sleep Environment

- **Comfortable Bedding**: Ensure your mattress and pillows are comfortable and supportive.

- **Dark and Quiet Room**: Keep your bedroom dark, quiet, and cool to create an optimal sleep environment. Use blackout curtains, earplugs, or a white noise machine if necessary.

- **Limit Electronic Devices**: Avoid screens (TV, smartphone, computer) at least an hour before bedtime, as the blue light can interfere with your sleep.

3. Pay Attention to Your Diet

- **Avoid Stimulants**: Limit caffeine and nicotine, especially in the hours leading up to bedtime, as they can disrupt your sleep.

- **Eat Light in the Evening**: Avoid heavy or large meals close to bedtime. Opt for a light snack if you're hungry in the evening.

4. Stay Active

- **Regular Exercise**: Engage in regular physical activity to promote better sleep. However, avoid vigorous exercise close to bedtime as it may interfere with your ability to fall asleep.

5. Manage Stress and Relax

- **Relaxation Techniques**: Practice relaxation techniques such as deep breathing, meditation, or progressive muscle relaxation to reduce stress and prepare your body for sleep.

- **Limit Naps**: If you need to nap, keep it short (20-30 minutes) and early in the day to avoid interfering with your nighttime sleep.

By incorporating regular exercise, managing stress effectively, and ensuring quality sleep, you can significantly reduce inflammation and improve your overall health. These lifestyle changes, combined with an anti-inflammatory diet, create a holistic approach to wellness that supports long-term health and vitality.

TIPS FOR DINING OUT AND SOCIAL EVENTS

Maintaining an anti-inflammatory lifestyle while dining out or attending social events can be challenging, but it's entirely possible with a little preparation and mindfulness. This chapter will provide practical tips and strategies to help you make healthy, anti-inflammatory choices in various social settings, ensuring you can enjoy these occasions without compromising your health goals.

Tips for Dining Out

1. **Plan Ahead**:

   - **Research Restaurants**: Look up menus online before choosing a restaurant to ensure they offer healthy, anti-inflammatory options. Many places provide nutritional information and ingredient lists.

   - **Call Ahead**: Don't hesitate to call the restaurant to ask about their ability to accommodate dietary restrictions and preferences.

2. **Make Smart Menu Choices**:

   - **Opt for Whole Foods**: Choose dishes that emphasize whole, unprocessed ingredients like vegetables, lean proteins, and whole grains.

   - **Avoid Fried Foods**: Opt for grilled, baked, steamed, or roasted options instead of fried foods.

- **Substitute Sides**: Swap out less healthy sides like French fries for vegetables, salads, or whole grains.

3. **Control Portions**:

   - **Share Meals**: Consider sharing an entrée with a friend or family member to avoid overeating.

   - **Order a Starter**: Sometimes, an appetizer or a combination of appetizers can make a healthy, balanced meal.

   - **Take Leftovers Home**: Don't feel obligated to finish large portions; ask for a to-go container to enjoy the rest later.

4. **Mindful Eating Practices**:

   - **Eat Slowly**: Take your time to savor each bite, which can help you enjoy your meal more and recognize when you're full.

   - **Avoid Distractions**: Focus on your food and company, rather than your phone or the restaurant's TV screens.

   - **Listen to Your Body**: Pay attention to your hunger and fullness cues to prevent overeating.

5. **Healthy Beverage Choices**:

   - **Water**: Stick to water, perhaps with lemon, to stay hydrated without added sugars.

- **Herbal Tea**: Opt for herbal tea or unsweetened beverages as an alternative to sugary drinks and alcohol.

Tips for Social Events

1. **Bring a Dish**:

   - **Potluck Style**: Offer to bring an anti-inflammatory dish to share. This ensures you have at least one healthy option available.

   - **Healthy Snacks**: Bring along some healthy snacks like nuts, fruit, or veggie sticks to share and enjoy.

2. **Eat Before You Go**:

   - **Healthy Pre-Meal**: Have a small, healthy meal or snack before attending an event. This way, you're less likely to overindulge in less healthy options.

3. **Focus on Socializing**:

   - **Engage in Conversation**: Shift your focus from the food to enjoying the company of friends and family.

   - **Activity-Based Events**: Suggest activities that don't revolve around food, such as playing games, going for a walk, or attending a cultural event.

4. **Manage Alcohol Consumption**:

- **Limit Alcohol**: Alcohol can be inflammatory, so limit your intake. Opt for red wine in moderation, which contains antioxidants, or choose non-alcoholic beverages.

- **Drink Water**: Alternate alcoholic drinks with water to stay hydrated and reduce overall alcohol consumption.

5. **Navigate Buffets Wisely**:

- **Survey the Options**: Take a moment to look at all the offerings before filling your plate. This helps you make more intentional choices.

- **Fill Up on Veggies**: Start with a large portion of vegetables and salads, and then add smaller portions of proteins and whole grains.

- **Watch Portions**: Use a smaller plate if available, and avoid going back for seconds unless you're truly still hungry.

6. **Communicate Your Needs**:

- **Host Communication**: If you feel comfortable, let your host know about your dietary preferences or restrictions ahead of time.

- **Be Polite and Grateful**: Express gratitude for the food offered, and politely decline items that don't fit your diet without drawing too much attention.

Strategies for Travel and Holidays

1. **Pack Snacks**:

    - **Healthy Options**: Bring along portable, anti-inflammatory snacks such as nuts, seeds, fruit, and whole-grain crackers.

    - **Stay Prepared**: Having healthy snacks on hand can help you avoid less healthy options at airports, rest stops, and hotels.

2. **Choose Accommodations with Kitchens**:

    - **Self-Catering**: When possible, stay in places that allow you to cook your own meals. This gives you control over your ingredients and meal preparation.

3. **Stay Hydrated**:

    - **Water Bottle**: Carry a refillable water bottle to ensure you stay hydrated and avoid sugary drinks.

4. **Stick to Your Routine**:

    - **Exercise and Sleep**: Try to maintain your regular exercise and sleep routines as much as possible while traveling. This helps keep your body balanced and reduces stress.

5. **Mindful Indulgence**:

   - **Special Treats**: Allow yourself to enjoy special treats in moderation. Savor them mindfully, and balance indulgences with healthier meals.

Building Resilience and Flexibility

1. **Practice Self-Compassion**:

   - **Be Kind to Yourself**: Recognize that it's okay to indulge occasionally and that one meal won't derail your health goals.

   - **Learn and Adjust**: Use any less-than-ideal eating experiences as learning opportunities for future situations.

2. **Set Realistic Expectations**:

   - **Balance and Enjoyment**: Aim for balance rather than perfection. Enjoy the social aspects of dining out and events without stressing over every food choice.

   - **Gradual Changes**: Incorporate small, sustainable changes over time rather than drastic, restrictive measures.

3. **Stay Connected to Your Goals**:

- **Remind Yourself**: Keep your health goals in mind when making food choices, and remember the benefits of an anti-inflammatory diet.

- **Visualize Success**: Visualize how good you feel when you make healthy choices, which can motivate you to stay on track.

By following these tips and strategies, you can navigate dining out and social events with confidence, making choices that align with your anti-inflammatory lifestyle while still enjoying the social and culinary experiences. Remember, the key is balance and mindfulness, allowing you to maintain your health goals without sacrificing enjoyment and connection.

INCORPORATING MINDFUL EATING PRACTICES

Mindful eating is an essential component of an anti-inflammatory lifestyle. It involves paying full attention to the experience of eating, recognizing physical hunger and satiety cues, and making conscious food choices that promote health and well-being. This chapter will guide you through the principles of mindful eating and provide practical tips for incorporating these practices into your daily routine.

Principles of Mindful Eating

1. **Awareness**:

   - Pay attention to your food, how it looks, smells, tastes, and feels.

   - Notice the colors, textures, and flavors of your meals.

   - Be present in the moment and avoid distractions like television or smartphones while eating.

2. **Hunger and Fullness Cues**:

   - Listen to your body's signals of hunger and fullness.

   - Eat when you're hungry and stop when you're satisfied, not when you're overly full.

   - Differentiate between physical hunger and emotional hunger.

3. **Non-Judgment**:

   - Approach eating with a non-judgmental attitude.

   - Avoid labeling foods as "good" or "bad." Instead, consider how they make you feel and their nutritional value.

   - Be kind to yourself and avoid guilt about your food choices.

4. **Savoring**:

   - Take the time to savor each bite.

   - Chew slowly and thoroughly to enjoy the full experience of eating.

   - Appreciate the effort that went into growing, preparing, and cooking your food.

Tips for Incorporating Mindful Eating Practices

1. **Create a Calm Eating Environment**:

   - Set up a peaceful, clutter-free space for meals.

   - Use soft lighting and play calming music if it helps you relax.

   - Make mealtime a special occasion by setting the table and eliminating distractions.

2. **Practice Gratitude**:

- Before eating, take a moment to express gratitude for your food.

- Reflect on the journey of your food from farm to table and appreciate everyone involved in its production.

3. **Start with Small Portions**:

- Serve yourself smaller portions to prevent overeating.

- You can always go back for more if you're still hungry.

4. **Engage Your Senses**:

- Take a few deep breaths before you start eating to center yourself.

- Observe the colors, shapes, and presentation of your food.

- Notice the aromas and anticipate the flavors.

5. **Slow Down**:

- Put your fork down between bites to slow your eating pace.

- Chew each bite thoroughly and savor the textures and flavors.

- Take small sips of water to cleanse your palate and extend your meal time.

6. **Listen to Your Body**:

- Check in with yourself halfway through your meal to assess your hunger level.

- Stop eating when you feel comfortably satisfied, not when you're stuffed.

- Pay attention to how different foods make you feel after eating.

7. **Avoid Multitasking**:

- Focus solely on eating during mealtimes.

- Avoid watching TV, working, or using your phone while you eat.

- Allow yourself to fully engage in the act of eating and enjoy the experience.

8. **Reflect on Your Eating Habits**:

- Keep a food journal to track what you eat, how much you eat, and how you feel before and after meals.

- Identify patterns and triggers for mindless eating, such as stress or boredom.

- Use this awareness to make more mindful food choices.

9. **Practice Self-Compassion**:

- Be gentle with yourself if you overeat or make less healthy food choices.

- Understand that mindful eating is a practice, and it's normal to have setbacks.

- Focus on progress, not perfection, and continue to make small, positive changes.

Benefits of Mindful Eating

Incorporating mindful eating practices into your lifestyle offers numerous benefits:

1. **Improved Digestion**:

- Eating slowly and chewing thoroughly aids digestion and nutrient absorption.

- Reduced stress while eating can also improve digestive function.

2. **Better Appetite Regulation**:

- Listening to hunger and fullness cues helps prevent overeating and supports healthy weight management.

- Mindful eating can help break the cycle of emotional eating.

3. **Enhanced Enjoyment of Food**:

- Being fully present during meals enhances the sensory experience of eating.

- You're more likely to enjoy and appreciate your food, leading to greater satisfaction.

4. **Greater Awareness of Food Choices**:

- Mindful eating encourages you to choose foods that nourish your body and make you feel good.

- You become more attuned to how different foods affect your energy, mood, and overall well-being.

5. **Reduced Stress and Anxiety**:

- Mindful eating promotes relaxation and reduces stress around food and eating.

- It can also improve your relationship with food, fostering a more positive and balanced approach.

By incorporating these mindful eating practices into your daily routine, you can transform your relationship with food, enhance your overall health, and support your journey towards an anti-inflammatory lifestyle. Mindful eating is not about following strict rules but about cultivating a deeper connection with your food and your body, leading to a more satisfying and nourishing eating experience.

CONCLUSION

As we come to the end of this journey through the realm of anti-inflammatory eating, it's essential to reflect on the key principles and practices we've explored together. Throughout this book, we've delved into the transformative power of embracing an anti-inflammatory lifestyle, understanding the profound impact of inflammation on our health, and discovering the array of nourishing foods that can help us combat inflammation and optimize our well-being.

We've learned about the foundational principles of an anti-inflammatory diet, from emphasizing whole, nutrient-rich foods to minimizing processed and inflammatory ingredients. We've explored the importance of mindful eating, meal planning, and preparation techniques to support our journey towards better health. We've celebrated the abundance of delicious and satisfying recipes that align with the principles of anti-inflammatory eating, nourishing our bodies and delighting our taste buds in equal measure.

But beyond the recipes and meal plans, the heart of this book lies in its commitment to empowering you, the reader, to take control of your health and embark on a path of lasting wellness. As you embrace the anti-inflammatory lifestyle, remember that every small step you take towards prioritizing your health is a powerful act of self-care and self-love.

Maintaining long-term success with the anti-inflammatory lifestyle is not just about what you eat, but how you live. It's about cultivating habits that nourish not only your body but also your mind and spirit. It's about finding joy and fulfillment in the journey towards better health, embracing balance, and honoring your body's unique needs.

So, as you continue on your anti-inflammatory journey, may you approach each day with intention, mindfulness, and gratitude. May you savor the nourishing meals you prepare, finding pleasure and satisfaction in every bite. And may you thrive, embracing the vitality and wellness that comes from honoring your body and embracing the anti-inflammatory lifestyle.

Here's to your health, happiness, and long-term success with the anti-inflammatory lifestyle Diet cookbook.

With warmest wishes,
Grace Mitchell

30-Days Anti-Inflammatory Meal Plan

Week 1

Day 1

- **Breakfast:** Berry Spinach Smoothie Bowl
- **Lunch:** Mediterranean Chickpea Salad
- **Snack:** Hummus with Cucumber Slices
- **Dinner:** Grilled Salmon with Quinoa and Asparagus

Day 2

- **Breakfast:** Overnight Oats with Blueberries and Chia Seeds
- **Lunch:** Thai Chicken Lettuce Wraps
- **Snack:** Roasted Chickpeas
- **Dinner:** Lentil and Vegetable Stew

Day 3

- **Breakfast:** Turmeric and Ginger Smoothie
- **Lunch:** Zucchini Noodles with Pesto and Cherry Tomatoes
- **Snack:** Greek Yogurt with Berries and Honey
- **Dinner:** Baked Cod with Sweet Potato and Brussels Sprouts

Day 4

- **Breakfast:** Quinoa Breakfast Porridge
- **Lunch:** Roasted Butternut Squash and Kale Salad
- **Snack:** Apple Slices with Almond Butter
- **Dinner:** Chicken and Vegetable Stir-Fry

Day 5

- **Breakfast:** Chia Pudding with Mango and Coconut
- **Lunch:** Garlic Lemon Shrimp with Zoodles
- **Snack:** Edamame with Sea Salt
- **Dinner:** Stuffed Portobello Mushrooms

Day 6

- **Breakfast:** Green Detox Smoothie
- **Lunch:** Spinach and Mushroom Quinoa
- **Snack:** Trail Mix with Nuts and Dried Fruit
- **Dinner:** Baked Salmon with Asparagus

Day 7

- **Breakfast:** Oatmeal with Flaxseeds and Berries
- **Lunch:** Quinoa and Black Bean Tacos
- **Snack:** Carrot and Celery Sticks with Tahini Dip
- **Dinner:** Turmeric Roasted Cauliflower and Chickpeas

Week 2

Day 8

- **Breakfast:** Avocado Toast with Cherry Tomatoes and Basil
- **Lunch:** Mediterranean Chickpea Salad
- **Snack:** Roasted Chickpeas
- **Dinner:** Baked Cod with Sweet Potato and Brussels Sprouts

Day 9

- **Breakfast:** Sweet Potato Hash with Spinach and Eggs
- **Lunch:** Garlic Lemon Shrimp with Zoodles
- **Snack:** Greek Yogurt with Berries and Honey
- **Dinner:** Lentil and Vegetable Stew

Day 10

- **Breakfast:** Spinach and Mushroom Egg Muffins
- **Lunch:** Zucchini Noodles with Pesto and Cherry Tomatoes
- **Snack:** Hummus with Cucumber Slices
- **Dinner:** Grilled Salmon with Quinoa and Asparagus

Day 11

- **Breakfast:** Banana Almond Butter Toast
- **Lunch:** Chicken and Vegetable Stir-Fry
- **Snack:** Apple Slices with Almond Butter
- **Dinner:** Stuffed Portobello Mushrooms

Day 12

- **Breakfast:** Pumpkin Spice Smoothie
- **Lunch:** Spinach and Mushroom Quinoa
- **Snack:** Roasted Chickpeas
- **Dinner:** Quinoa and Black Bean Tacos

Day 13

- **Breakfast:** Coconut Almond Granola
- **Lunch:** Roasted Butternut Squash and Kale Salad
- **Snack:** Edamame with Sea Salt
- **Dinner:** Baked Cod with Sweet Potato and Brussels Sprouts

Day 14

- **Breakfast:** Berry Spinach Smoothie Bowl
- **Lunch:** Mediterranean Chickpea Salad
- **Snack:** Carrot and Celery Sticks with Tahini Dip
- **Dinner:** Turmeric Roasted Cauliflower and Chickpeas

Week 3

Day 15

- **Breakfast:** Overnight Oats with Blueberries and Chia Seeds
- **Lunch:** Thai Chicken Lettuce Wraps
- **Snack:** Trail Mix with Nuts and Dried Fruit
- **Dinner:** Grilled Salmon with Quinoa and Asparagus

Day 16

- **Breakfast:** Turmeric and Ginger Smoothie
- **Lunch:** Zucchini Noodles with Pesto and Cherry Tomatoes
- **Snack:** Greek Yogurt with Berries and Honey
- **Dinner:** Chicken and Vegetable Stir-Fry

Day 17

- **Breakfast:** Quinoa Breakfast Porridge
- **Lunch:** Garlic Lemon Shrimp with Zoodles
- **Snack:** Roasted Chickpeas
- **Dinner:** Lentil and Vegetable Stew

Day 18

- **Breakfast:** Chia Pudding with Mango and Coconut
- **Lunch:** Spinach and Mushroom Quinoa
- **Snack:** Apple Slices with Almond Butter
- **Dinner:** Stuffed Portobello Mushrooms

Day 19

- **Breakfast:** Green Detox Smoothie
- **Lunch:** Mediterranean Chickpea Salad
- **Snack:** Hummus with Cucumber Slices
- **Dinner:** Baked Salmon with Asparagus

Day 20

- **Breakfast:** Oatmeal with Flaxseeds and Berries
- **Lunch:** Quinoa and Black Bean Tacos
- **Snack:** Greek Yogurt with Berries and Honey
- **Dinner:** Turmeric Roasted Cauliflower and Chickpeas

Day 21

- **Breakfast:** Avocado Toast with Cherry Tomatoes and Basil
- **Lunch:** Chicken and Vegetable Stir-Fry
- **Snack:** Edamame with Sea Salt
- **Dinner:** Baked Cod with Sweet Potato and Brussels Sprouts

Week 4

Day 22

- **Breakfast:** Sweet Potato Hash with Spinach and Eggs
- **Lunch:** Spinach and Mushroom Quinoa
- **Snack:** Carrot and Celery Sticks with Tahini Dip
- **Dinner:** Lentil and Vegetable Stew

Day 23

- **Breakfast:** Spinach and Mushroom Egg Muffins
- **Lunch:** Garlic Lemon Shrimp with Zoodles
- **Snack:** Trail Mix with Nuts and Dried Fruit
- **Dinner:** Stuffed Portobello Mushrooms

Day 24

- **Breakfast:** Banana Almond Butter Toast
- **Lunch:** Zucchini Noodles with Pesto and Cherry Tomatoes
- **Snack:** Roasted Chickpeas
- **Dinner:** Grilled Salmon with Quinoa and Asparagus

Day 25

- **Breakfast:** Pumpkin Spice Smoothie
- **Lunch:** Mediterranean Chickpea Salad
- **Snack:** Greek Yogurt with Berries and Honey
- **Dinner:** Chicken and Vegetable Stir-Fry

Day 26

- **Breakfast:** Coconut Almond Granola
- **Lunch:** Spinach and Mushroom Quinoa
- **Snack:** Apple Slices with Almond Butter
- **Dinner:** Quinoa and Black Bean Tacos

Day 27

- **Breakfast:** Berry Spinach Smoothie Bowl
- **Lunch:** Thai Chicken Lettuce Wraps
- **Snack:** Hummus with Cucumber Slices
- **Dinner:** Baked Cod with Sweet Potato and Brussels Sprouts

Day 28

- **Breakfast:** Overnight Oats with Blueberries and Chia Seeds
- **Lunch:** Garlic Lemon Shrimp with Zoodles
- **Snack:** Greek Yogurt with Berries and Honey
- **Dinner:** Lentil and Vegetable Stew

Day 29

- **Breakfast:** Turmeric and Ginger Smoothie
- **Lunch:** Zucchini Noodles with Pesto and Cherry Tomatoes
- **Snack:** Roasted Chickpeas
- **Dinner:** Grilled Salmon with Quinoa and Asparagus

Day 30

- **Breakfast:** Quinoa Breakfast Porridge
- **Lunch:** Spinach and Mushroom Quinoa
- **Snack:** Apple Slices with Almond Butter
- **Dinner:** Chicken and Vegetable Stir-Fry